NEUROSCIENCE RESEARCH PROGRESS

VASOPRESSIN

MECHANISMS OF ACTION, PHYSIOLOGY AND SIDE EFFECTS

NEUROSCIENCE RESEARCH PROGRESS

Additional books in this series can be found on Nova's website under the Series tab.

Additional e-books in this series can be found on Nova's website under the e-book tab.

ENDOCRINOLOGY RESEARCH AND CLINICAL DEVELOPMENTS

Additional books in this series can be found on Nova's website under the Series tab.

Additional e-books in this series can be found on Nova's website under the e-book tab.

NEUROSCIENCE RESEARCH PROGRESS

VASOPRESSIN

MECHANISMS OF ACTION, PHYSIOLOGY AND SIDE EFFECTS

LEONZIO GALELLA
EDITOR

NOVINKA

New York

For permission to use material from this book please contact us:
Telephone 631-231-7269; Fax 631-231-8175
Web Site: http://www.novapublishers.com

Library of Congress Cataloging-in-Publication Data

ISBN: 978-1-62417-311-0
Library of Congress Control Number: 2012952354

Published by Nova Science Publishers, Inc. † New York

CONTENTS

PREFACE

Vasopressin is a hormone involved in water balance and osmoregulation. It is produced by the hypothalamus and released by the neuro-pituitary. In this book, the authors discuss the mechanisms of action, physiology and side effects of vasopressin. Topics include the study of the role of vasopressin in hypothalamo-pituitary-adrenocortical (HPA) axis regulation; vasopressin used in both adult and pediatric vasodilatory shock and cardiac arrest; the therapeutic potential and challenges of modulating myometrial smooth muscle tone through the vasopressin V1A receptor; the efficacy of vasoactive medications in acute variceal bleeds; and the reproductive and metabolic responses of desert adapted common spiny male mice to vasopressin treatment.

Chapter 1 – The authors environment can be considered as a set of stressors. Adaptation to them is indispensable to life. However, overloading the hypothalamo-pituitary-adrenocortical (HPA) axis, one of the major components of adaptation, often leads to stress-related diseases. Therefore understanding the mechanisms of stress processes is highly important. The hypothalamic component of the HPA axis consists of corticotropin-releasing hormone (CRH) and vasopressin, with a questionable contribution of the latter. The natural vasopressin knockout Brattleboro strain is a good tool for the stress-free study of the role of vasopressin in HPA axis regulation. Data from this strain was compared to knockout mice, vasopressin-antiserum and V1b receptor antagonist studies. In adult Brattleboro rats the vasopressin-deficiency did not influence the resting levels as well as the development of chronic stress state. However, the CRH-supporting effect of vasopressin was observable after different acute stress situations, where the exact role depended on the nature of the stressor encountered. In contrast, vasopressin had more crucial role in the regulation of the adrenocorticotropin (ACTH, the hypophyseal level of the HPA axis) secretion during the perinatal age, which was observable during a wide range of relevant physiological stress processes. The dissociation between ACTH and corticosterone secretion (the next, adrenal level of the HPA axis) was surprising. The vasopressin deficiency resulted in higher corticosterone levels than expected based on the low stressor-induced ACTH secretion, therefore an ACTH-independent adrenal gland regulation can be assumed. There was no obvious difference in the HPA axis regulatory role of vasopressin between the two genders. The authors can conclude that vasopressin plays a more important role in the stress-axis regulation during early development, than we previously thought.

Chapter 2 – Vasopressin has been used in both adult and pediatric vasodilatory shock and cardiac arrest. The evidence in this area is primarily adult based, while pediatric specific data is more limited. The rationale for vasopressin in shock is based on the following: 1) it reverses the key mechanisms responsible for pathologic vasodilatation and catecholamine resistance, 2) despite its potent systemic vasoconstrictor properties, vasopressin has concurrent organ-specific vasodilator effects that may result in preserved vital organ perfusion; 3) vasopressin influences multiple other hormone responses which may modulate hypothalamic-pituitary axis dysfunction and cellular immune response during septic shock; and 4) vasopressin insufficiency, and an increased sensitivity to the pressor effects of exogenous vasopressin has been demonstrated in both adults and perhaps children with septic shock.

There are to date a total of 40 published pediatric studies evaluating the use of vasopressin in shock, reporting on a collective total of only 642 children. 35 of these studies are in shock, and 5 studies are in cardiac arrest. The vast majority of studies are case reports or case series. Only 2 of these studies are randomized controlled trials (RCT) – one of which was a multi-centred, double-blind RCT of arginine vasopressin in 69 patients vasodilatory shock, while the other was an open-label 58 patient RCT of terlipressin in catecholamine-resistant septic shock While there may be some evidence of short-term benefits with no increased risk of adverse effects, there has been no demonstrable superiority of vasopressin over traditional vasoactive agents on patient important outcomes such as survival, in children with catecholamine-refractory shock and cardiopulmonary arrest. As a result, vasopressin is not currently recommended as a first line vasoactive agent in pediatric patients with hemodynamic instability. The mortality rate amongst children with shock remains unacceptably high, ranging from 15-70%. As a result, these challenges and controversies rationalize the importance of ongoing prospective research on a potential role for vasopressin in the setting of pediatric shock.

Chapter 3 – Arginine vasopressin plays a key role in the regulation of diverse physiological processes in the cardiovascular, renal, uterine and CNS systems. Abnormal release or activation of vasopressin receptors appears to contribute to the disease pathogenesis and physiology of a number of conditions including polycystic kidney disease, congestive heart failure, septic shock and depression, especially.

In recent years, both improved biophysical techniques as well as the discovery of potent and selective vasopressin ligands have helped facilitate a better understanding of the critical receptors involved in these disease processes. The authors will outline the role of vasopressin in the regulation of normal myometrial smooth muscle contraction during menstruation and parturition as well as the consequences of inappropriate activation leading to dysmenorrhoea and early labour.

Chapter 4 – Vasoactive medications such as vasopressin, somatostatin and their analogues are commonly used for the treatment of acute variceal bleeding. Vasoactive medications have been used for over thirty years and management has improved with better endoscopic therapies and the use of antibiotics prophylactically. Even with such a long history, the risks and benefits of the use of vasoactive medications continue to be debated. In this article the authors explore the evidence behind the efficacy of these medications.

Chapter 5 – Changes in day length (photoperiod) can serve as an important signal for the coming breeding season for mammals inhabiting predictable ecosystems in temperate zones. In unpredictable desert ecosystems, photoperiod changes are not a sufficient signal to predict the optimal time of breeding. Therefore, integration of various environmental cues should determine which species will be adapted to breed at the right time and to survive in xeric environments. In regards the authors asked the following question: What are the environmental cues and their mechanism used by xeric adapted small mammals for reproduction timing? The driving force in desert ecosystems is water and the intervals between episodes of water input into the ecosystem vary and in some years there may be no input. It has been suggested that water availability can serve as a reliable cue for reproduction.

Vasopressin (VP), a hormone involved in water balance and osmoregulation is produced by the hypothalamus and released by the neuro-pituitary. VP secretion levels increase in response to elevated plasma osmolarity, representing water shortage. VP receptors are found in the reproductive tract. The different effects of VP on metabolism and reproduction make it candidate for mediating the transmission of environmental signals to the reproductive system of desert adapted rodents. The authors tested the metabolic and reproductive response of males from a desert adapted population of *A. cahirinus* to VP treatment under three week acclimation to two different photoperiod regimes short (SD- 8L:16D) and long (LD-16L:8D). The results of the authors study show that VP treatment *per se*, caused a significant ($p<0.05$) decrease of testosterone level in SD-acclimated males. VP treatment caused an increase in FFA release of SD-acclimated males but not in LD-males. In addition, response was assessed from changes in mRNA receptor gene expression of VP (AVP) and aldosterone (nr3c2) in testis and white adipose tissue (WAT) of treated groups, compared with their control. VP treatment resulted in a decrease of VP receptor gene expression, in LD-acclimated male testis. VP caused a significant decrease in aldosteron receptor mRNA expression in SD-acclimated males, in testis, but caused its elevation in WAT. These results support the idea that water availability in the habitat may affect breeding through effects of VP, directly, on the testis, or indirectly through effects on WAT. These findings also support previous knowledge that different physiological systems could be integrated by a single hormonal signal.

In: Vasopressin
Editor: Leonzio Galella

ISBN: 978-1-62417-311-0

Chapter 1

AN UNFAIRLY UNDERVALUED PARTICIPANT OF THE STRESS PROCESSES: THE VASOPRESSIN

János Varga and Dóra Zelena*
Institute of Experimental Medicine,
Hungarian Academy of Sciences,
Budapest, Hungary

ABSTRACT

Our environment can be considered as a set of stressors. Adaptation to them is indispensable to life. However, overloading the hypothalamo-pituitary-adrenocortical (HPA) axis, one of the major components of adaptation, often leads to stress-related diseases. Therefore understanding the mechanisms of stress processes is highly important. The hypothalamic component of the HPA axis consists of corticotropin-releasing hormone (CRH) and vasopressin, with a questionable contribution of the latter. The natural vasopressin knockout Brattleboro strain is a good tool for the stress-free study of the role of vasopressin in HPA axis regulation. Data from this strain was compared to knockout mice, vasopressin-antiserum and V1b receptor antagonist studies. In adult Brattleboro rats the vasopressin-deficiency did not influence the resting

* Corresponding author: Dóra Zelena, Institute of Experimental Medicine, Hungarian Academy of Sciences. 1083 Budapest. Szigony 43. Hungary. Tel.: +36-1-210-9400/124. Fax: +36-1-210-9951. E-mail: zelena.dora@koki.mta.hu.

levels as well as the development of chronic stress state. However, the CRH-supporting effect of vasopressin was observable after different acute stress situations, where the exact role depended on the nature of the stressor encountered. In contrast, vasopressin had more crucial role in the regulation of the adrenocorticotropin (ACTH, the hypophyseal level of the HPA axis) secretion during the perinatal age, which was observable during a wide range of relevant physiological stress processes. The dissociation between ACTH and corticosterone secretion (the next, adrenal level of the HPA axis) was surprising. The vasopressin deficiency resulted in higher corticosterone levels than expected based on the low stressor-induced ACTH secretion, therefore an ACTH-independent adrenal gland regulation can be assumed. There was no obvious difference in the HPA axis regulatory role of vasopressin between the two genders. We can conclude that vasopressin plays a more important role in the stress-axis regulation during early development, than we previously thought.

Keywords: Chronic stress, acute stress, perinatal period, sex, catecholamine

INTRODUCTION

The term stress is commonly used, but difficult to define. It is used generally when we feel that everything becomes too much - we are overloaded and wonder whether we really can cope with the pressures placed upon us. Any challenge or a threat to our well-being is a stress. However, without any stress at all we probably would die. Stress is the body's way to handle a challenge and preparing to meet a tough situation with focus, strength, stamina, and heightened alertness. In that sense stress is good, helps the adaptation. However, long-term stressful situations can produce a lasting stress that is hard on people. The body senses continued pressure and remains slightly activated and continues to pump out extra stress hormones over an extended period. This wears out the body's reserves, weakens the body's immune system, thus can undermines both our mental and physical health (Simonton and Matthews-Simonton, 1981). Several disorders can be connected with stress like stomach ulceration (Lam et al., 1995), high blood pressure (Sparrenberger et al., 2009) or diabetes mellitus (Lehman et al., 1991). Stress regulates also the fertility (Demyttenaere et al., 1991). On the list of reasons of mental disorders stress became a prominent issue. Most important stress-related psychiatric disorders are anxiety and depression (Checkley, 1996), schizophrenia and posttraumatic stress disorder (Cohen,

1993). They may also lead to a "vicious circle", as these disorders themselves serve as stressors.

According to Hans Selye, the father of the stress concept, the activation of the hypothalamo-pituitary-adrenocortical (HPA) axis is one of the main background mechanisms of adaptation (Selye, 1975) (Figure 1). The central part of this axis consists of two neurohormones, corticotropin-releasing hormone (CRH) and arginine vasopressin (AVP) released from the nucleus paraventricularis hypothalami (PVN) into the portal blood (Antoni, 1993).

They act synergistically on the anterior pituitary to stimulate adrenocorticotropin (ACTH) synthesis from the proopiomelanocortin (POMC) gene and its release (Lutz-Bucher et al., 1980; Rivier and Vale, 1983). ACTH reaches the adrenal gland through general circulation, where it stimulates the glucocorticoid synthesis and release.

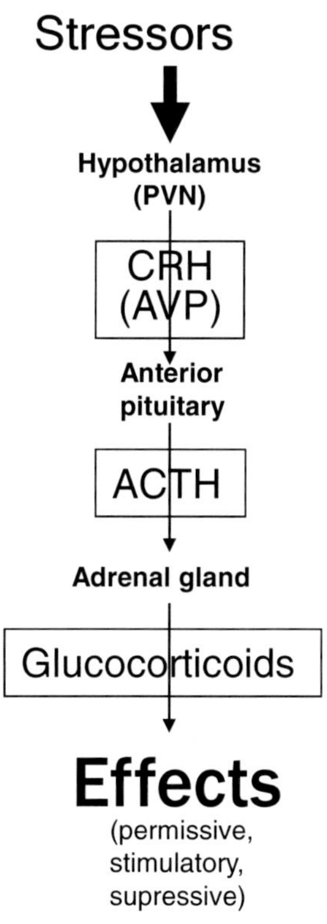

Figure 1. Elements of the stress axis. PVN- nucleus paraventricularis hypothalami; CRH - corticotropin releasing hormone; AVP – arginine vasopressin; ACTH- adrenocorticotropin.

Glucocorticoids (mainly cortisol in humans and corticosterone (B) in rodents) are the effector molecules of the axis with permissive (expression of various proteins), stimulatory (carbohydrate metabolism) and suppressive (anti-inflammatory, immunosuppressive, negative feedback) actions (Sapolsky et al., 2000).

Following its identification in 1954, AVP was thought to be the principal regulator of the ACTH release (Du Vigneaud, 1954). After identification of CRH, and the domination of Dale's Law (one neuron/one transmitter) (Dale, 1935) the role of AVP in stress regulation was waned. There was no doubt that AVP stimulated ACTH secretion but only in high, non-physiological concentrations (Buckingham, 1982). A landmark was the idea of Dallman (Dallman, 1993) and Aguilera (Aguilera, 1994) with a prominent AVP regulation of the HPA axis during chronic stress. According to Engelmann (Engelmann et al., 2004) during eustress AVP may influence the ACTH secretion through different pathways (Figure 2): (1) AVP colocalized with CRH in the parvocellular cells of the PVN is released into the portal circulation and reaches the anterior lobe via long portal vessels. (2) AVP is released en passant from axons of magnocellular neurons at the level of the median eminence. (3) AVP is secreted from axon terminals in the posterior pituitary into short portal vessels, which supply the anterior lobe. (4) AVP is secreted from axon terminals in the posterior pituitary into the general blood circulation. (5) Local release of AVP from dendrites and somata affects the activity of the parvo/magnocellular neurons directly (autofeedback) or indirectly (e.g., via modulation of afferents and/or blood supply and/or via the action of other, co-expressed neuropeptides). During distress, an additional level is proposed: (6) The prolonged hyperactivity of the HPA axis results in a sustained somato-dendritic release of AVP from magnocellular neurons within the PVN. This AVP may partially diffuse out of the PVN to reach remote limbic brain areas, including the septum thereby altering the interpretation of the stressor, thus the entire stress response. Later studies did not fully confirm the heuristic view of AVPerg HPA axis regulation during chronic/excessive stress. Nevertheless the question arose, what could be the physiological role of AVP in stress regulation. The present review will focus on different aspects of this question.

The problem with stress studies is that any handling (even control saline injection) is an additional stressor. Therefore, knockout animals seem to be preferable tools for stress research. In that sense, the spontaneous AVP mutant Brattleboro rat seems to be a good tool.

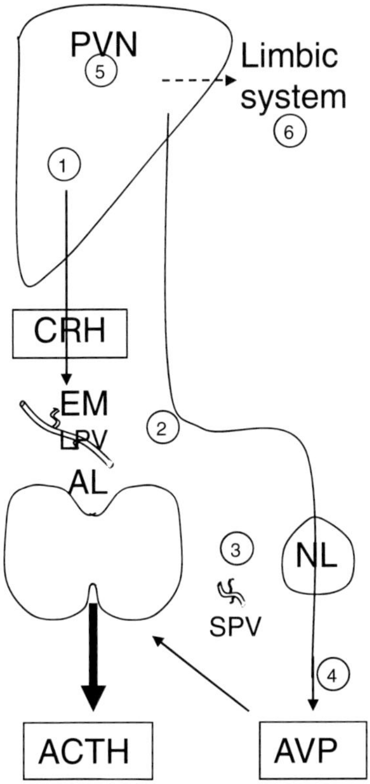

Figure 2. Possible site of effects of vasopressin on ACTH secretion. PVN- nucleus paraventricularis hypothalami, CRH-corticotropin releasing hormone, EM- eminentia mediana, AL- anterior lobe of the pituitary, NL- neural lobe of the pituitary, LPV-long portal vessels, SPV-short portal vessels, ACTH- adrenocorticotropin, AVP-vasopressin (For details see text).

This strain was discovered in 1961 in West Brattleboro, Vermont as a spontaneous mutation in the Long Evans strain (Valtin, 1982). These rats carry a single base deletion in the neurophysin region of the AVP gene, and in the homozygous (AVP-) animal this recessive mutation results in an inability to process the gene product to AVP, while the heterozygous (AVP+) rats have normal AVP function (Schmale et al., 1984). As these rats are littermates, heterozygous animals are appropriate controls (Bohus and de Wied, 1998). In the following data on the Brattleboro animals will be compared with other tools, like knockout mice, AVP antiserum, and V1b receptor antagonists (like SSR-149415 or the Org V1bR antagonist), as the main pituitary AVP receptor belongs to the V1b subtype (Serradeil-Le Gal et al., 2002b; Serradeil-Le Gal et al., 2005; Spiga et al., 2009a; Spiga et al., 2009b).

It is known in general that the effects of hormones could be different in the two genders, and it was proved also for AVP. E.g. desmopressin, an AVP agonist has different antidiuretic effect in men than in women (Juul et al., 2011). Moreover, gender-specific differences in basal and stress-induced HPA secretion are detectable already at birth (Patchev et al., 1999). To explore gender differences we studied the HPA axis of both male and female Brattleboro rats.

Basal Levels

Theoretically AVP may be an important component in the maintenance of the resting activity of the HPA axis. Despite an early report on lower basal ACTH and B levels (Buckingham, 1982) our studies on Brattleboro rats did not confirm a damped HPA axis among rest (Figure 3). Moreover, even the diurnal variation in ACTH and B secretion was not influenced by the genotype (Zelena et al., 2009a).

This was true not only in male but also in female animals and not only for the plasma levels but also on the ACTH precursor POMC mRNA level in the anterior lobe of the pituitary. The only significant difference was detectable at the hypothalamic level, where the CRH mRNA level was lower in both genders. This was surprising as we expected a compensatory elevation and not a reduction. Nevertheless previous studies confirmed a lower CRH content in the hypothalamus (Buckingham, 1982).

One might argue that during the decades of breeding the Brattleboro colony changed and therefore not reflect any more the HPA axis regulatory role of AVP, as in 1982 the resting stress-hormone levels were lower in AVP-deficient Brattleboro animals, but not after 2005. However, this is unlikely as there was no difference between the genotypes in the V1b receptor knockout mice, either (Lolait et al., 2007a).

Immunoneutralization studies in rats found no role of AVP in the maintenance of the resting levels, too (Ono et al., 1985; Tilders et al., 1985). Basal secretion and diurnal variations of ACTH and cortisol were unaltered in the group of anti-AVP-immunized sheep, as well (Guillaume et al., 1992). Both the SSR-149415 and the Org V1bR antagonist had no effect on basal ACTH and B secretion, or on the pulsatility of the B secretion (Craighead et al., 2008; Spiga et al., 2009b; Zelena et al., 2011).

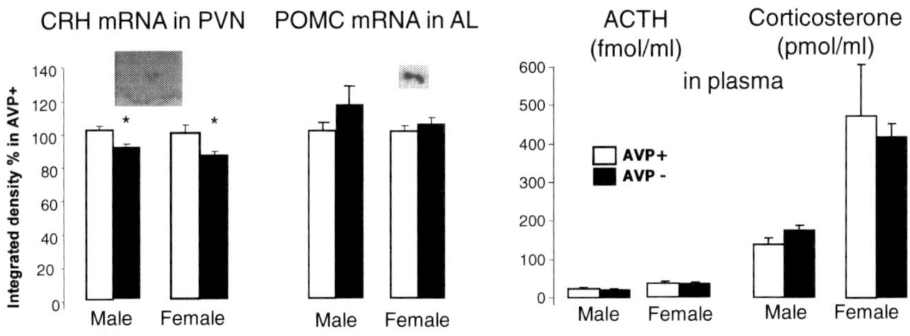

Figure 3. Resting hypothalamo-pituitary-adrenocortical axis parameters in Brattleboro rats. CRH - corticotropin releasing hormone; PVN - nucleus paraventricularis hypothalami; POMC - proopiomelanocortin; AL - anterior lobe of the pituitary; ACTH - adrenocorticotropin; AVP - vasopressin. *$p<0.05$ vs. AVP+.

Therefore it is more likely, that the development of methodology for the detection of hormones is responsible for the discrepancy between previous and present results, and indeed AVP has no major role in the maintenance of resting HPA axis activity.

Acute Stress

To have a clear picture we conducted a detailed analysis on Brattleboro rats using wide range of acute stressors (Zelena et al., 2009a). We have shown that the AVP is important for stressor-induced ACTH secretion during most acute stimuli. However, its contribution to B secretion was more variable. Therefore three category could have been formulated: 1) stressors with decreased ACTH and B responses (volume load, morphine injection, aggressive contact, restraint); 2) stressors with a decreased ACTH response but no change in B (novelty, elevated plus maze, lipopolysaccharide injection, ip hypertonic saline injection, forced swim, hypoglycaemia, anaphylaxis, ulcerogen cold restraint); 3) stimuli without a change in ACTH or B response (social avoidance, footshock, ether inhalation).

A highly repeatable and robust change was found with iv. egg-white-induced anaphylactoid reaction and Actrapid (rapid insulin) induced hypoglycaemic stress in both genders (Figure 4). Although it was restricted only for the ACTH levels and the B levels were unaffected.

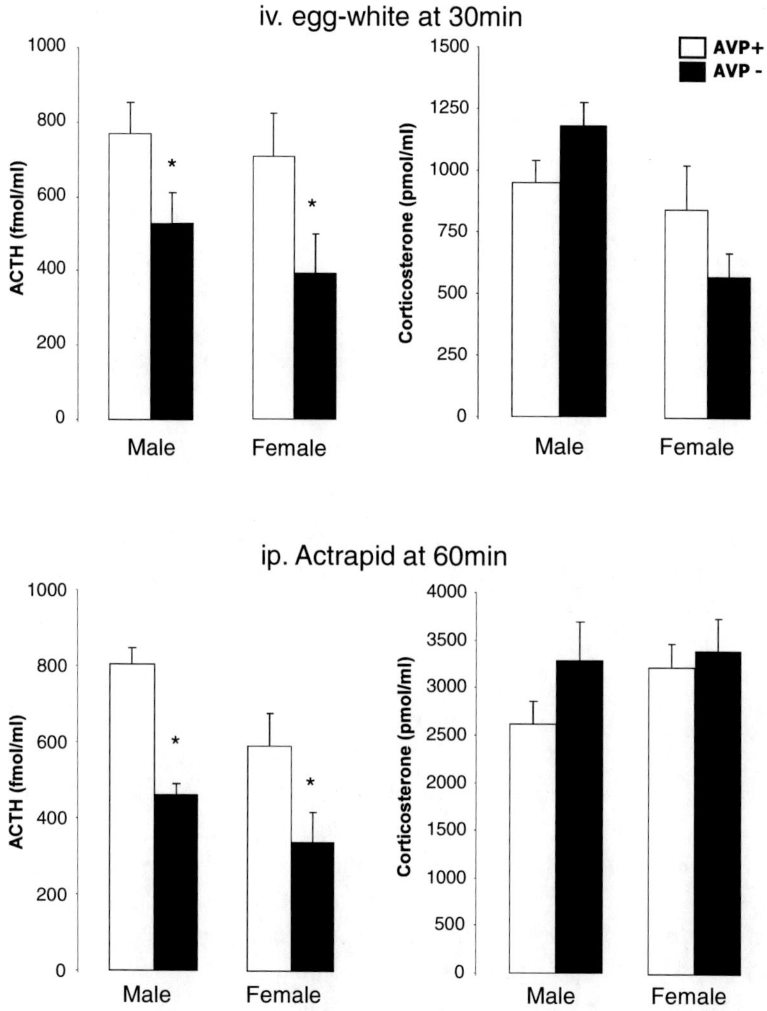

Figure 4. Acute stress in Brattleboro rats. Plasma adrenocorticotropin (ACTH) and corticosterone levels 30 min after intravenous (iv) injection of a diluted egg-white solution (Foldes et al., 2000) or 60min after intraperitoneal (ip) injection of 3NE Actrapid (rapid insulin (Zelena et al., 2009a)) measured from cannulated or decapitated animals, respectively. *p<0.05 vs. AVP+.

There is a wide range of studies on the role of AVP during acute stimuli. Aggressive contact-induced release of ACTH and B was similar in wild type and V1bR knockout mice, but the hypoglycemia-, lipopolysaccharide-, forced swim- and ethanol-intoxication-induced elevations were significantly diminished and restraint- (30 min) induced elevation was in one report normal, while in an other smaller (Lolait et al., 2007a; Lolait et al., 2007b; Roper et al., 2010; Tanoue et al., 2004). Immunoneutralization studies revealed a role of AVP in restraint-, formalin- and ether stress- induced ACTH elevation (Ono et al., 1985; Tilders et al., 1985). ACTH and cortisol responses both to insulin-induced hypoglycemia and isolation-restraint stress and CRH injection were significantly reduced in anti-AVP-immunized sheep compared to those in controls (Guillaume et al., 1992). The selective, nonpeptide V1bR antagonist (SSR149415) was able to diminish the restraint-induced ACTH increase by 50% (Serradeil-Le Gal et al., 2002a) and inhibited the response to ether exposure but failed to inhibit the HPA axis during forced swim (Ramos et al., 2006). Another V1b antagonist (Org) diminished the restraint-, forced swimg- and lipopolysaccharide-induced ACTH changes without affecting the noise stress-induced changes and the B levels (Roper et al., 2010; Spiga et al., 2009b). More precisely the restraint-induced B elevation was smaller in male V1bR knockout as well as Org V1bR antagonist treated mice compared to appropriate controls, but not in females (Roper et al., 2010).

We can conclude that AVP is important, although not exclusive, for the stressor-induced ACTH secretion, but has subtle effect on B secretion independently from the gender. As B is the effective endhormone of the HPA axis and there is a clear dissociation between ACTH and B secretion two questions arose: (1) what is the regulator of the B secretion? (2) what is the role of stressor-induced ACTH secretion?

ACTH-Independent Regulation of the Corticosterone Secretion

Hypothalamic and pituitary lesions with the absence of ACTH lead to adrenal atrophy and adrenocortical insufficiency, which could be restored by ACTH administration. Based on these clear-cut anatomical, physiological and clinical observations, it has become generally accepted that adrenocortical glucocorticoid secretion is exclusively linked to pituitary ACTH release. There is no doubt on the importance of ACTH in the maintenance of the integrity of the adrenal gland, thereby basal B secretion. However, in acute stress situations in Brattleboro rats it has been found that the B changes followed the ACTH plasma levels changes just in a small part of the experimental series. Although ACTH and B levels at a given time point could dissociate for various reason, in Brattleboro rats we closed out the possibility of the temporal lag (by serial blood sampling), of the enhanced adrenal gland sensitivity to ACTH (by *in vitro* studies) and the differences in B binding capacity (as we measured all and not just the effective free B concentration) (Zelena et al., 2009a; Zelena et al., 2011). Moreover, similar dissociation was found with a V1bR antagonist (Org) (Spiga et al., 2009b) and in the V1bR knockout mice (Stewart et al., 2008). In addition, relevant physiological and clinical paradigms exist that demonstrate a dissociation between ACTH and B levels (Bornstein et al., 2008). These findings raise the possibility that other peripheral mediators are involved and act directly on the adrenal gland. These results support the existence of ACTH-independent glucocorticoid secretion (Bornstein et al., 2008) that was formulated first in the theory of para-adenohypophyseal neuroendocrine regulation (Elifanov et al., 1988). ACTH-independent mechanisms seem to have an important role in fine-tuning and modulating the highly sensitive adrenal stress system to adapt its response appropriately to physiological needs.

A large number of neuropeptides, neurotransmitters, opioids, growth factors, cytokines, adipokines and even bacterial ligands are capable of modulating adrenal glucocorticoid release independently of pituitary ACTH. Obvious candidates are the catecholamines, as the adrenal medulla, secreting adrenaline, is in close vicinity to the cortex, and splanchnic nerve innervation may modulate glucocorticoid secretion via catecholaminerg receptors, too (Bornstein et al., 1990; Edwards, 1997; Holzwarth et al., 1987). All catecholamine receptors were found on the adrenal cortex (Sundaresan et al., 1987), however, the beta receptors were suggested to be the most important ones (Holzwarth et al., 1987; Mazzocchi et al., 1997). As previous studies used mostly *in vitro* incubation systems or agonist, the *in vivo*, physiological role of endogenous catecholamines is unclear. Therefore, in a previous study we have used the 10-day-old AVP-deficient rat pup as a model organism, where stressors may induce B rise without previous ACTH elevation (Makara et al., 2012). This is a unique model to study possible *in vivo* mechanisms that regulate directly the glucocorticoid secretion of the adrenal cortex. Indeed, we have shown with a hypoglycemic stressor that propranolol (a beta-receptor antagonist) significantly reduced the stressor-induced changes. We can add, however, that even higher doses of propranolol could not completely block the stressor-induced rise, thereby it is quite probable that other factors are simultaneously involved.

THE EXTRA-ADRENAL ROLE OF ACTH

Based upon other results showing an enhanced ACTH release accompanied by minor changes in glucocorticoid secretion another conclusion could also be drawn. Namely that ACTH - secreted during stress – is likely to have some other role(s) beside the glucocorticoid secretion regulation (for a review see (Zelena and Makara, 2011)).

Resting ACTH secretion is an important contributor not only to the maintenance of the integrity of the adrenal gland, but also to many aspects of its development. ACTH regulates the steroid synthesis and release in the adrenal gland, first of all synthesis of glucocorticoids, but also the adrenal androgens and mineralocorticoids are affected. The synthesis of steroids can be enhanced in other steroidogenic tissues, too (Horvath et al., 1986; Varga et al., 1986). Already in the 60s researcher of our Institute established that ACTH might influence not only the adrenal, but also the ovarian blood flow (Stark and Varga, 1968). The cardiovascular effects include blood pressure elevation (Bertolini, 1995) and enhancement of local blood flow (Stark and Varga, 1968), together with an effect on the salt-water homeostasis (especially natriuresis) (Gruber et al., 1984). Similarly to glucocorticoids, ACTH has also a direct anti-inflammatory action both on the thymus and on the circulating lymphocytes (Brod and Hood, 2011; Catania et al., 2011; Montero-Melendez et al., 2011). ACTH regulates the carbohydrate and lipid homeostasis in the brain, liver, pancreas and brown adipose tissue (Lesault et al., 1991; Lewis and Matthews, 1968; Spirovski et al., 1975). Exogenous melanocortins may markedly influence the behavior, although the role of endogenous melanocortins is doubtful in this respect (Bertolini et al., 2009).

These extra-adrenal effects of ACTH are worth to consider not only for research purposes, but also during the increasing number of diagnostic and therapeutic usage of ACTH, e.g. infant spasm (Mikati et al., 2002), epilepsy (Gayatri et al., 2007), lipid-lowering activity (Thorisdottir et al., 2009).

CHRONIC STRESS

Chronic stress seems to be more important for the development of different disorders, in case the organism is overloaded. A shift to AVP predominance in the CRH/AVP ratio in the PVN after chronic stimulation suggested a prominent role of AVP in the maintenance the HPA axis activity during chronic stress (Aguilera, 1994; Dallman, 1993; Lightman et al., 2002; Ma and Lightman, 1998). These assumptions originated from studies on adrenalectomized animals, which – due to the missing negative feedback – have similarly activated HPA axis as during chronic stress (Makino et al., 1995). Later studies with chronic stressors confirmed these shift in rats with repeated restraint, repeated insulin injections, chronic psychosocial stress, chronic food deprivation, adjuvant-induced arthritis, as well as in spontaneous autoimmune-disease developing mice (Chowdrey et al., 1995; De Goeij et al., 1992a; De Goeij et al., 1992b; Hwang and Guntz, 1997; Makara et al., 2004; Pinnock and Herbert, 2001; Sakic et al., 1999).

As HPA axis regulatory AVP came basically from the PVN first we used PVN lesions to dissect the role of this hypothalamic nucleus in chronic stress-induced somatic and HPA axis changes. When we compared 3 different kinds of chronic stressors applied for one or two weeks the relative importance of the PVN was found to be different in the three models (Table 1).

Twenty four hours after 7 days daily 60 min restraint both the POMC mRNA level in the anterior lobe of the pituitary and the plasma B level were significantly higher compared to control, but these changes were prevented in PVN lesioned rats, suggesting a prominent role of this hypothalamic nucleus in the regulation (Zelena et al., 2003).

On the other hand, the presence of PVN was not necessary for the development of hyperactivity of the HPA axis in adjuvant-induced arthritis model (Makara et al., 2001). In the case of this immune challenge a direct activation of the ACTH secretion at the pituitary level can be supposed through enhanced presence of stimulatory cytokines (IL-1, IL-2, IL-11) (Cai et al., 2006; Jones et al., 1993; Prickett et al., 2000; van der Meer et al., 1996). Moreover, IL-1beta and IL-6 can also stimulate the pituitary ACTH secretion through AVP-release from the neurointermediate lobe (Yasin et al., 1994)

Table 1. Effect of PVN lesion on the pituitary and adrenal level of the hypothalamo-pituitary-adrenal axis after chronic stress

	Effect of PVN lesion on		Main centrum	Reference
	POMC mRNA	Plasma B levels		
7R	+	+	PVN	Zelena et al. 2003
AA	-	-	Hypophysis	Makara et al. 2001
DM	+	-	Adrenal gland	Zelena et al. 2006

7R- repeated restraint daily 60 min; AA- adjuvant-induced arthritis for 14 days; DM- streptozotocin-induced diabetes mellitus for 14 days.

An interesting stimulatory process was observed in streptozotocin-induced diabetes mellitus rats (Zelena et al., 2006a). Here, despite the missing POMC mRNA elevation in the anterior pituitary after PVN lesion the plasma B levels were still elevated. This suggests a direct metabolic regulation of the B release at the adrenal gland level, which is highly independent from the stressor-induced ACTH release.

Based upon the PVN lesion studies we could have supposed that AVP will not have had a regulatory role on B secretion in diabetes mellitus. However, several facts suggested that AVP may indeed participate in the process. (1) AVP from other than PVN origin might regulate the ACTH secretion (Figure 2) (Engelmann et al., 2004) (2) magnocellular cells of the supraoptic nucleus contains more AVP than the PVN (Rhodes et al., 1981) (3) AVP, acting via V1 receptors located in adrenals, exerts a stimulating effects on adrenal regeneration (Trejter et al., 2005). (4) During dehydration, elevated plasma AVP can stimulate the production of B by the adrenal, independently of ACTH (Wotus et al., 2003). (5) AVP is synthesized and secreted by chromaffin cells either present in the medulla or scattered throughout the cortex of the adrenal gland (Gallo-Payet and Guillon, 1998). AVP receptors are also present; they belong to V1aR on the cortex, while on cromaffin cells to V1bR subtype.

Using Brattleboro rats we found that AVP does not play a crucial role in HPA axis regulation during diabetes mellitus-induced chronic stress (Zelena et al., 2006a; Zelena et al., 2006b). In contrast, the role of AVP was more important during acute restraint, however, it was restricted only to the ACTH regulation.

Therefore next we studied if AVP has a prominent role during repeated restraint-induced HPA axis changes, as it could have been supposed based on PVN lesion experiments. The body weight reduction developed in both gender during the 14day daily 1h restraint, with smaller diminution in AVP-deficient females (Figure 5). The thymus were smaller in both chronically stressed genders compared to controls, but the AVP-deficiency was not protective, on the contrary, in AVP-deficient male rats the thymus involution was even more pronounced. The adrenal gland hyperplasia was detectable only in males. In females the relative weight of the adrenal gland was significantly higher than in males, perhaps that was the reason, while no further elevation to chronic stressors was detectable. Interestingly, in this experiment the resting plasma concentration of B was not higher in females than in males (Figure 6) despite the larger adrenals, although the combination of different experiments shows an elevated resting B levels in females compared to males (Figure 3).

Chronic stress was able to enhance the ACTH content of the anterior lobe, as well as the plasma B levels, but only in males. The plasma levels of ACTH was not elevated due to the fact, that this peptide hormone could be stored and the plasma levels therefore does not necessarily reflect an enhanced synthesis rate.

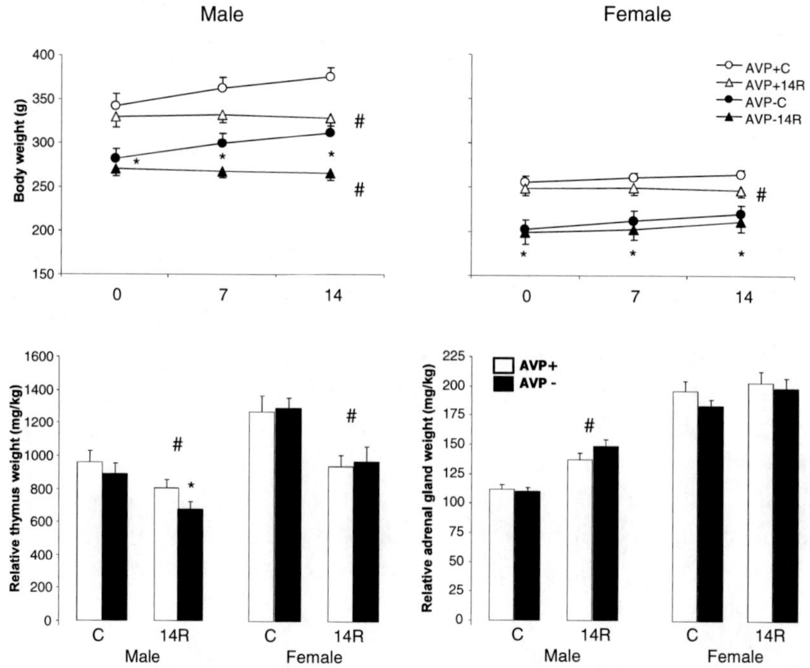

Figure 5. Somatic parameters after repeated restraint in Brattleboro rats. Rats were stressed by daily 60 min restaint (Zelena et al., 2004) and decapitated among rest on day 15., 24h after the last stressor. C - control, unstressed animals; 14R- chronically stressed group. *p<0.05 vs. AVP+; #p<0.05 vs. C.

On the contrary, the steroid hormone B cannot be stored, therefore its enhanced synthesis rate is easily detected at the periphery, in the blood. Two other pituitary hormones, beta-endorphine and prolactin plasma levels were not influenced by repeated retraint. However, the AVP-deficiency significantly enhanced the first (beta-endorphine) and reduced the later (prolactin). As beta-endorphine is also a POMC derivate, it is not a surprise that its plasma level is not influenced by chronic stressor, although previous studies reported an enhancement in its releasable pool after repeated footshock (Young and Akil,

1985). The enhanced beta-endorphine levels in AVP-deficient animals can contribute to changes in pain sensitivity after chronic stressors (Bradesi et al., 2009). Previous studies with repeated restraint was unable to find any alteration in resting prolactin levels (Adler and Sokol, 1982; Sokol and Zimmerman, 1982; Zelena et al., 2003). Prolactin stimulates the secretion of AVP as part of the maternal adaptations facilitating parturition and lactation (Vega et al., 2010). On the other hand AVP administration can stimulate prolactin secretion (Sharshar and Annane, 2008). Recent findings with reduced prolactin levels in Brattleboro rats support that AVP is important for the maintenance of resting prolactin secretion (Figure 6).

In the Brattleboro strain adjuvant injections do not lead to development of arthritis. Therefore it was impossible to study the role of AVP in this disease-model. We used repeated short periods of morphine withdrawals instead (Houshyar et al., 2003). Although the typical somatic (body weight and thymus reduction and adrenal gland hypertrophy) and HPA axis parameters (POMC mRNA level elevation in the anterior lobe of the pituitary and resting B plasma level enhancement) developed, but we could not detect any differences between the genotypes in the Brattleboro rats (Domokos et al., 2008). In contrast, we have found that AVP played a prominent role in morphine treatment and withdrawal-induced acute hormone changes. These differences could be indeed important as stress responsive AVP/V1b receptor systems may be critical components of the neural circuitry underlying the aversive emotional consequences of drug withdrawal, as well as the effect of negative emotional states on drug-seeking behavior (Zhou et al., 2008).

In V1bR knockout mice the AVP was found to be important only for ACTH but not B regulation during 14 day repeated restraint stress (Lolait et al., 2007a). The Org V1bR antagonist prevented the exaggerated ACTH response to noise after repeated restraint, however, had no effect on the development of chronic stress state or on B levels (Spiga et al., 2009a). On the contrary, another V1bR antagonist, the SSR149415 was ineffective to modulate the changed (diminished or increased) acute response after repeated restraint in rats (Chen et al., 2008). Despite the ineffectiveness on HPA axis parameters SSR149415 completely prevented chronic water stress-induced visceral hyperalgesia (Bradesi et al., 2009). This suggests that brain AVP might have important regulatory role on the emotions and behavior, which is independent from its HPA axis regulatory effects. Indeed, a vast body of evidence supports the involvement of AVP in anxiety and depression (Frank and Landgraf, 2008; Scott and Dinan, 2002; Zelena, 2009).

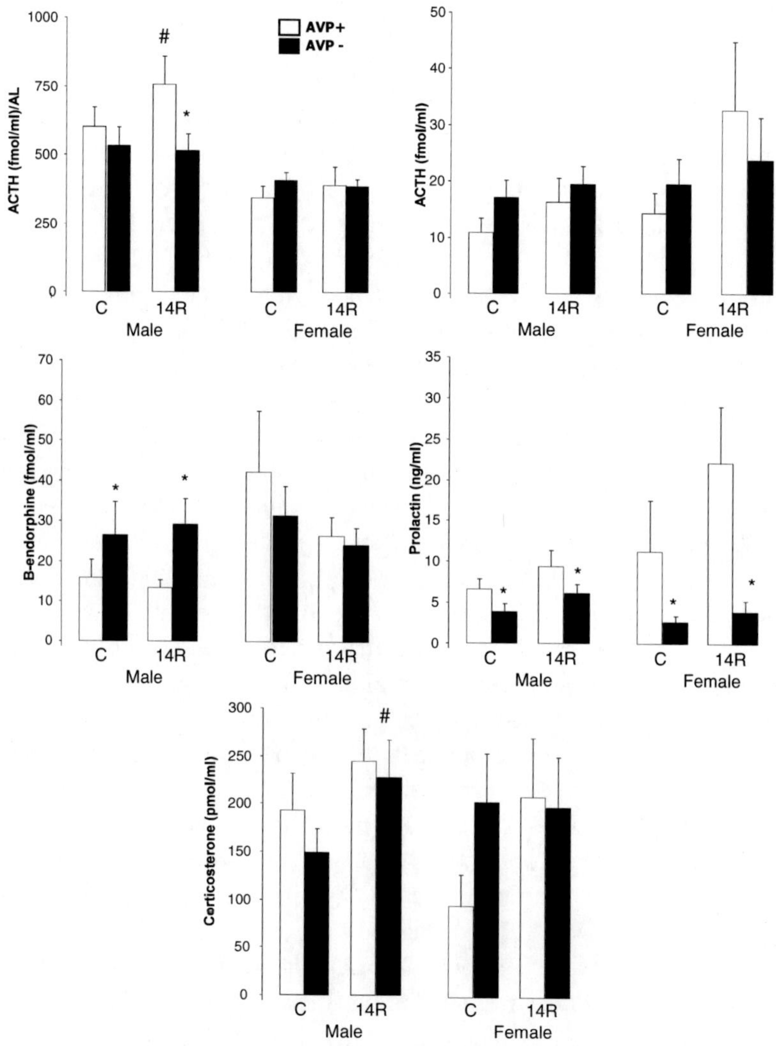

Figure 6. Hormone levels after repeated restraint in Brattleboro rats. Rats were stressed by daily 60 min restaint (Zelena et al., 2004) and decapitated among rest on day 15., 24h after the last stressor. ACTH - adrenocorticotropin, AL- anterior lobe of the pituitary; C - control, unstressed animals; 14R- chronically stressed group. *p<0.05 vs. AVP+; #p<0.05 vs. C.

Taken together AVP in not indispensable for the development of chronic stress state, however, it may have a role in the maintenance of acute stress reactivity in a chronically stressed organism.

PERINATAL PERIOD

As the development of compensatory mechanism is increasing with age we decided to study the role of AVP in HPA axis regulation during the perinatal period, too (Zelena et al., 2008a; Zelena et al., 2008b; Zelena et al., 2009b; Zelena et al., 2011). The hypothesis that during the perinatal period AVP may be the main regulator of the HPA axis was tested (Avishai-Eliner et al., 1995; Levine, 2002).

Single Hypnorm (μ-opiate agonist) injection is a potent stimulus of the HPA axis of the newborn (Barna et al., 1993) (Figure 7).

The ACTH elevation was absolutely missing from the 10-day-old AVP-deficient pups independently from the gender. On the contrary, B secretion was even more pronounced in AVP-deficient animals. In females the maximal ACTH secretion was smaller than in males, but there was no difference in B secretion. We got similar results with three other types of stressor, namely after 24h maternal separation, single (10 min) or repeated (70 min) ether inhalation and bacterial lipopolysaccharide (LPS) injection (Zelena et al., 2008b; Zelena et al., 2011). Thus, the hypothesis that AVP is the principal regulator of the ACTH secretion during the perinatal period has been supported by these studies. Development of compensation is less likely in a 10-day-old animal than in adults. Indeed, both the pituitary oxytocin (structural, anatomical and partly functional 'twin' of AVP) content (Zelena et al., 2011) and the CRH mRNA level in the PVN (Zelena et al., 2008b) were lower in AVP-deficient pups compared to their heterozygous littermates.

Moreover, the other important regulatory system, the sympatho adrenomedulary axis, does not seem to be overactivated in di/di pups (Zelena et al., 2008a), despite the enhanced catecholamine plasma levels (Kvetnansky et al., 1990) as well as pituitary and brain content in adults (Holzbauer et al., 1980). Theoretically it would be possible that the higher resting B levels of AVP-deficient pups would restrain the ACTH secretion by negative feedback.

To exclude this we have used both a V1bR antagonist (SSR-149415) (Zelena et al., 2011) and an AVP antiserum (Makara et al., 2012) in control +/+ pups to inhibit the lipopolisaccharide-induced HPA axis activity with the same results (dissociation of ACTH and B) without resting B elevation. In fetal sheep there is also a direct anatomical evidence for AVP innervation of the adrenal gland (Hoffman et al., 1989).

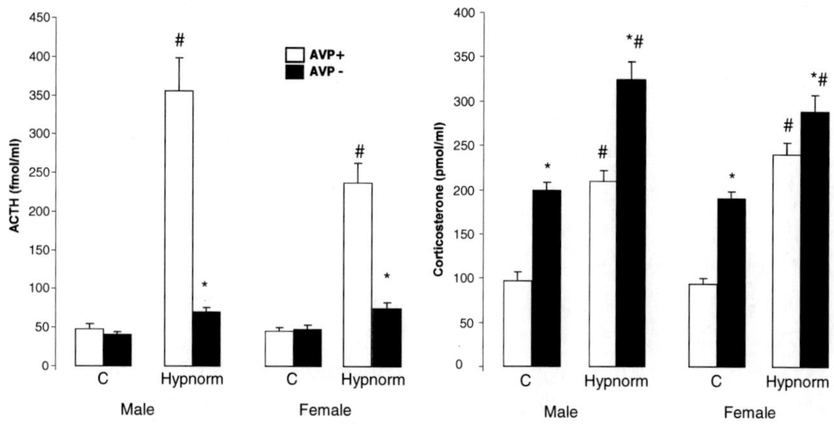

Figure 7. Hypnorm-induced stress-hormone changes in 10-day-old Brattleboro pups. Sixty min after an intraperitoneal injection of 1 μl/g fentanyl-fluanisone combination (Hypnorm) or saline pups were decapitated and hormone levels were measured by radioimmunoassay (Zelena et al., 2008b). C - control, saline injected. *$p<0.05$ vs. AVP+; #$p<0.05$ vs. C.

All these results supported the idea that AVP is an important regulator of ACTH release in neonatal animals. The dissociation of ACTH and B secretion was reviewed previously.

CONCLUSION

Based upon the above data we can conclude that the role of AVP in HPA axis regulation

- is limited upon rest, but might has a role in the maintenance the basal prolactin secretion
- during acute stress is stressor specific
- is not needed for the development of chronic stress, but in some case AVP is important for the maintenance of acute reactivity in a chronically stressed animal
- more important during the perinatal period (restricted to ACTH)
- is similarly important in the two genders

Our conclusions do not seem to be influenced by compensatory factors in Brattleboro rats as most of the results were confirmed using V1bR antagonists (chronic stress (Chen et al., 2008), acute stress (Craighead et al., 2008; Serradeil-Le Gal et al., 2003; Spiga et al., 2009b), perinatal period (Zelena et al., 2011)).

ACKNOWLEDGMENT

Supported by grants NN 71629 from OTKA, Hungary.

REFERENCES

Adler, R.A., Sokol, H.W., 1982. Prolactin and growth hormone in the unstressed Brattleboro rat. *Ann. N Y Acad. Sci.* 394, 607-13.

Aguilera, G., 1994. Regulation of pituitary ACTH secretion during chronic stress. *Front Neuroendocrinol.* 15, 321-50.

Antoni, F.A., 1993. Vasopressinergic control of pituitary adrenocorticotropin secretion comes of age. *Front Neuroendocrinol.* 14, 76-122.

Avishai-Eliner, S., Yi, S.J., Newth, C.J., Baram, T.Z., 1995. Effects of maternal and sibling deprivation on basal and stress induced hypothalamic-pituitary-adrenal components in the infant rat. *Neurosci. Lett.* 192, 49-52.

Barna, I., Acs, Z., Koenig, J.I., 1993. Effects of Hypnorm (fentanyl) on ACTH/beta-endorphin levels in plasma, pituitary and brain of 10-day old rats. *Life Sci.* 52, 1417-24.

Bertolini, A., 1995. The opioid/anti-opioid balance in shock: a new target for therapy in resuscitation. *Resuscitation.* 30, 29-42.

Bertolini, A., Tacchi, R., Vergoni, A.V., 2009. Brain effects of melanocortins. *Pharmacol. Res.* 59, 13-47.

Bohus, B., de Wied, D., 1998. The vasopressin deficient Brattleboro rats: a natural knockout model used in the search for CNS effects of vasopressin. *Prog. Brain Res.* 119, 555-73.

Bornstein, S.R., Ehrhart-Bornstein, M., Scherbaum, W.A., Pfeiffer, E.F., Holst, J.J., 1990. Effects of splanchnic nerve stimulation on the adrenal cortex may be mediated by chromaffin cells in a paracrine manner. *Endocrinology.* 127, 900-6.

Bornstein, S.R., Engeland, W.C., Ehrhart-Bornstein, M., Herman, J.P., 2008. Dissociation of ACTH and glucocorticoids. *Trends Endocrinol Metab*. 19, 175-80.

Bradesi, S., Martinez, V., Lao, L., Larsson, H., Mayer, E.A., 2009. Involvement of vasopressin 3 receptors in chronic psychological stress-induced visceral hyperalgesia in rats. *Am. J. Physiol Gastrointest Liver* Physiol. 296, G302-9.

Brod, S.A., Hood, Z.M., 2011. Ingested (oral) ACTH inhibits EAE. *J. Neuroimmunol.* 232, 131-5.

Buckingham, J.C., 1982. Potentiation of hypothalamic corticotropin releasing activity by vasopressin: studies in the Brattleboro rat. *Ann. N Y Acad. Sci.* 394, 580-6.

Cai, X., Wong, Y.F., Zhou, H., Liu, Z.Q., Xie, Y., Jiang, Z.H., Bian, Z.X., Xu, H.X., Liu, L., 2006. Manipulation of the induction of adjuvant arthritis in Sprague-Dawley rats. *Inflamm Res*. 55, 368-77.

Catania, A., Lonati, C., Sordi, A., Carlin, A., Leonardi, P., Gatti, S., 2011. The melanocortin system in control of inflammation. *ScientificWorldJournal.* 10, 1840-53.

Checkley, S., 1996. The neuroendocrinology of depression and chronic stress. *Br. Med. Bull.* 52, 597-617.

Chen, J., Young, S., Subburaju, S., Sheppard, J., Kiss, A., Atkinson, H., Wood, S., Lightman, S., Serradeil-Le Gal, C., Aguilera, G., 2008. Vasopressin does not mediate hypersensitivity of the hypothalamic pituitary adrenal axis during chronic stress. *Ann. N Y Acad. Sci.* 1148, 349-59.

Chowdrey, H.S., Larsen, P.J., Harbuz, M.S., Jessop, D.S., Aguilera, G., Eckland, D.J., Lightman, S.L., 1995. Evidence for arginine vasopressin as the primary activator of the HPA axis during adjuvant-induced arthritis. *Br. J. Pharmacol.* 116, 2417-24.

Cohen, C.I., 1993. Poverty and the course of schizophrenia: implications for research and policy. *Hosp. Community Psychiatry*. 44, 951-8.

Craighead, M., Milne, R., Campbell-Wan, L., Watson, L., Presland, J., Thomson, F.J., Marston, H.M., Macsweeney, C.P., 2008. Characterization of a novel and selective V1B receptor antagonist. *Prog. Brain Res*. 170, 527-35.

Dale, H., 1935. Pharmacology and Nerve-endings (Walter Ernest Dixon Memorial Lecture): (Section of Therapeutics and Pharmacology). *Proc. R Soc. Med.* 28, 319-32.

Dallman, M.F., 1993. Stress update Adaptation of the hypothalamic-pituitary-adrenal axis to chronic stress. *Trends Endocrinol Metab*. 4, 62-9.

De Goeij, D.C., Binnekade, R., Tilders, F.J., 1992a. Chronic stress enhances vasopressin but not corticotropin-releasing factor secretion during hypoglycemia. *Am. J. Physiol*. 263, E394-9.

De Goeij, D.C., Dijkstra, H., Tilders, F.J., 1992b. Chronic psychosocial stress enhances vasopressin, but not corticotropin-releasing factor, in the external zone of the median eminence of male rats: relationship to subordinate status. *Endocrinology*. 131, 847-53.

Demyttenaere, K., Nijs, P., Evers-Kiebooms, G., Koninckx, P.R., 1991. Coping, ineffectiveness of coping and the psychoendocrinological stress responses during in-vitro fertilization. *J. Psychosom. Res*. 35, 231-43.

Domokos, A., Mergl, Z., Barna, I., Makara, G.B., Zelena, D., 2008. Congenital vasopressin deficiency and acute and chronic opiate effects on hypothalamo-pituitary-adrenal axis activity in Brattleboro rats. *J. Endocrinol*. 196, 113-21.

Du Vigneaud, V., 1954. Hormones of the posterior pituitary gland: oxytocin and vasopressin. *Harvey Lect*. 50, 1-26.

Edwards, A.V., 1997. Aspects of autonomic and neuroendocrine function. *Equine. Vet. J. Suppl*. 109-17.

Elifanov, A.V., Polenov, A.L., Belen'kii, M.A., Kuzik, V.V., 1988. [Morphofunctional research on the interrenal gland of the frog Rana temporaria following arginine vasotocin administration]. *Zh. Evol. Biokhim. Fiziol*. 24, 740-4.

Engelmann, M., Landgraf, R., Wotjak, C.T., 2004. The hypothalamic-neurohypophysial system regulates the hypothalamic-pituitary-adrenal axis under stress: an old concept revisited. *Front Neuroendocrinol*. 25, 132-49.

Foldes, A., Nemethy, Z., Szalay, O., Kovacs, K.J., 2000. Anaphylactoid reactions activate hypothalamo-pituitary-adrenocortical axis: comparison with endotoxic reactions. *Brain Res. Bull*. 52, 573-9.

Frank, E., Landgraf, R., 2008. The vasopressin system--from antidiuresis to psychopathology. *Eur. J. Pharmacol*. 583, 226-42.

Gallo-Payet, N., Guillon, G., 1998. Regulation of adrenocortical function by vasopressin. *Horm. Metab. Res*. 30, 360-7.

Gayatri, N.A., Ferrie, C.D., Cross, H., 2007. Corticosteroids including ACTH for childhood epilepsy other than epileptic spasms. *Cochrane Database Syst. Rev*. CD005222.

Gruber, K.A., Klein, M.C., Hutchins, P.M., Buckalew, V.M., Jr., Lymangrover, J.R., 1984. Natriuretic and hypertensive activities reside in a fragment of ACTH. *Hypertension*. 6, 468-74.

Guillaume, V., Conte-Devolx, B., Magnan, E., Boudouresque, F., Grino, M., Cataldi, M., Muret, L., Priou, A., Figaroli, J.C., Oliver, C., 1992. Effect of chronic active immunization with antiarginine vasopressin on pituitary-adrenal function in sheep. *Endocrinology*. 130, 3007-14.

Hoffman, G.E., McDonald, T., Figueroa, J.P., Nathanielsz, P.W., 1989. Neuropeptide cells and fibers in the hypothalamus and pituitary of the fetal sheep: comparison of oxytocin and arginine vasopressin. *Neuroendocrinology*. 50, 633-43.

Holzbauer, M., Sharman, D.F., Godden, U., Mann, S.P., Blatchford, D., Laverty, R., Jarvis, L.G., 1980. Observations on pituitary and cerebral catecholamines in Brattleboro rats. *Med. Biol.* 58, 25-32.

Holzwarth, M.A., Cunningham, L.A., Kleitman, N., 1987. The role of adrenal nerves in the regulation of adrenocortical functions. *Ann. N Y Acad. Sci.* 512, 449-64.

Horvath, E., Varga, B., Stark, E., 1986. Stimulation of progesterone production by adrenocorticotropic hormone and prostaglandin E2 in rat luteal cells. *Biol. Reprod.* 35, 44-8.

Houshyar, H., Gomez, F., Manalo, S., Bhargava, A., Dallman, M.F., 2003. Intermittent morphine administration induces dependence and is a chronic stressor in rats. *Neuropsychopharmacology*. 28, 1960-72.

Hwang, B.H., Guntz, J.M., 1997. Downregulation of corticotropin-releasing factor mRNA, but not vasopressin mRNA, in the paraventricular hypothalamic nucleus of rats following nutritional stress. *Brain Res. Bull.* 43, 509-14.

Jones, T.H., Kennedy, R.L., Justice, S.K., Price, A., 1993. Interleukin-1 stimulates the release of interleukin-6 from cultured human pituitary adenoma cells. *Acta Endocrinol. (Copenh)*. 128, 405-10.

Juul, K.V., Klein, B.M., Sandstrom, R., Erichsen, L., Norgaard, J.P., 2011. Gender difference in antidiuretic response to desmopressin. *Am. J. Physiol. Renal Physiol.* 300, F1116-22.

Kvetnansky, R., Jezova, D., Oprsalova, Z., Foldes, O., Michajlovskij, N., Dobrakovova, M., Lichardus, B., Makara, G.B., 1990. Regulation of the sympathetic nervous system by circulating vasopressin. *Adv. Exp. Med. Biol.* 274.

Lam, S.K., Hui, W.M., Shiu, L.P., Ng, M.M., 1995. Society stress and peptic ulcer perforation. *J. Gastroenterol. Hepatol.* 10, 570-6.

Lehman, C.D., Rodin, J., McEwen, B., Brinton, R., 1991. Impact of environmental stress on the expression of insulin-dependent diabetes mellitus. *Behav. Neurosci.* 105, 241-5.

Lesault, A., Elchinger, B., Desbals, B., 1991. Circadian variations and extraadrenal effect of ACTH on insulinemia in rabbit. *Horm. Metab. Res.* 23, 461-4.

Levine, S., 2002. Regulation of the hypothalamic-pituitary-adrenal axis in the neonatal rat: the role of maternal behavior. *Neurotox. Res.* 4, 557-564.

Lewis, G.P., Matthews, J., 1968. The mobilization of free fatty acids from rabbit adipose tissue in situ. *Br. J. Pharmacol.* 34, 564-78.

Lightman, S.L., Windle, R.J., Ma, X.M., Harbuz, M.S., Shanks, N.M., Julian, M.D., Wood, S.A., Kershaw, Y.M., Ingram, C.D., 2002. Hypothalamic-pituitary-adrenal function. *Arch. Physiol. Biochem.* 110, 90-3.

Lolait, S.J., Stewart, L.Q., Jessop, D.S., Young, W.S., 3rd, O'Carroll, A.M., 2007a. The hypothalamic-pituitary-adrenal axis response to stress in mice lacking functional vasopressin V1b receptors. *Endocrinology.* 148, 849-56.

Lolait, S.J., Stewart, L.Q., Roper, J.A., Harrison, G., Jessop, D.S., Young, W.S., 3rd, O'Carroll, A.M., 2007b. Attenuated stress response to acute lipopolysaccharide challenge and ethanol administration in vasopressin V1b receptor knockout mice. *J. Neuroendocrinol.* 19, 543-51.

Lutz-Bucher, B., Koch, B., Mialhe, C., Briaud, B., 1980. Involvement of vasopressin in corticotropin-releasing effect of hypothalamic median eminence extract. *Neuroendocrinology.* 30, 178-82.

Ma, X.M., Lightman, S.L., 1998. The arginine vasopressin and corticotrophin-releasing hormone gene transcription responses to varied frequencies of repeated stress in rats. *J. Physiol.* 510 (Pt 2), 605-14.

Makara, G.B., Harbuz, M.S., Coventry, T.L., Jessop, D.S., Zelena, D., Lightman, S.L., 2001. The effect of hypothalamic lesions on hypothalamo-pituitary-adrenal axis activity and inflammation in adjuvant-induced arthritis. Stress. 4, 25-37.

Makara, G.B., Mergl, Z., Zelena, D., 2004. The role of vasopressin in hypothalamo-pituitary-adrenal axis activation during stress: an assessment of the evidence. *Ann. N Y Acad. Sci.* 1018, 151-61.

Makara, G.B., Varga, J., Barna, I., Pinter, O., Klausz, B., Zelena, D., 2012. The vasopressin-deficient brattleboro rat: lessons for the hypothalamo-pituitary-adrenal axis regulation. *Cell Mol. Neurobiol.* 32, 759-66.

Makino, S., Smith, M.A., Gold, P.W., 1995. Increased expression of corticotropin-releasing hormone and vasopressin messenger ribonucleic acid (mRNA) in the hypothalamic paraventricular nucleus during repeated stress: association with reduction in glucocorticoid receptor mRNA levels. *Endocrinology*. 136, 3299-309.

Mazzocchi, G., Gottardo, G., Nussdorfer, G.G., 1997. Catecholamines stimulate steroid secretion of dispersed fowl adrenocortical cells, acting through the beta-receptor subtype. *Horm. Metab. Res*. 29, 190-2.

Mikati, M.A., Lepejian, G.A., Holmes, G.L., 2002. Medical treatment of patients with infantile spasms. *Clin. Neuropharmacol*. 25, 61-70.

Montero-Melendez, T., Patel, H.B., Perretti, M., 2011. Role of melanocortin receptors in the regulation of gouty inflammation. *Curr. Rheumatol. Rep*. 13, 138-45.

Ono, N., Bedran de Castro, J., Khorram, O., McCann, S.M., 1985. Role of arginine vasopressin in control of ACTH and LH release during stress. *Life Sci.* 36, 1779-86.

Patchev, V.K., Hayashi, S., Orikasa, C., Almeida, O.F., 1999. Ontogeny of gender-specific responsiveness to stress and glucocorticoids in the rat and its determination by the neonatal gonadal steroid environment. *Stress*. 3, 41-54.

Pinnock, S.B., Herbert, J., 2001. Corticosterone differentially modulates expression of corticotropin releasing factor and arginine vasopressin mRNA in the hypothalamic paraventricular nucleus following either acute or repeated restraint stress. *Eur. J. Neurosci*. 13, 576-84.

Prickett, T.C.R., Inder, W.J., Evans, M.J., Donald, R.A., 2000. Interleukin-1 potentiates basal and AVP-stimulated ACTH secretion in vitro the role of CRH pre-incubation. *Horm. Metab. Res*. 32, 350-4.

Ramos, A.T., Troncone, L.R., Tufik, S., 2006. Suppression of adrenocorticotrophic hormone secretion by simultaneous antagonism of vasopressin 1b and CRH-1 receptors on three different stress models. *Neuroendocrinology*. 84, 309-16.

Rhodes, C.H., Morrell, J.I., Pfaff, D.W., 1981. Immunohistochemical analysis of magnocellular elements in rat hypothalamus: distribution and numbers of cells containing neurophysin, oxytocin, and vasopressin. *J. Comp. Neurol*. 198, 45-64.

Rivier, C., Vale, W., 1983. Interaction of corticotropin-releasing factor and arginine vasopressin on adrenocorticotropin secretion in vivo. *Endocrinology*. 113, 939-42.

Roper, J.A., Craighead, M., O'Carroll, A.M., Lolait, S.J., 2010. Attenuated stress response to acute restraint and forced swimming stress in arginine vasopressin 1b receptor subtype (Avpr1b) receptor knockout mice and wild-type mice treated with a novel Avpr1b receptor antagonist. *J. Neuroendocrinol.* 22, 1173-80.

Sakic, B., Laflamme, N., Crnic, L.S., Szechtman, H., Denburg, J.A., Rivest, S., 1999. Reduced corticotropin-releasing factor and enhanced vasopressin gene expression in brains of mice with autoimmunity-induced behavioral dysfunction. *J. Neuroimmunol.* 96, 80-91.

Sapolsky, R.M., Romero, L.M., Munck, A.U., 2000. How do glucocorticoids influence stress responses? Integrating permissive, suppressive, stimulatory, and preparative actions. *Endocr. Rev.* 21, 55-89.

Schmale, H., Ivell, R., Breindl, M., Darmer, D., Richter, D., 1984. The mutant vasopressin gene from diabetes insipidus (Brattleboro) rats is transcribed but the message is not efficiently translated. *Embo. J.* 3, 3289-93.

Scott, L.V., Dinan, T.G., 2002. Vasopressin as a target for antidepressant development: an assessment of the available evidence. *J. Affect Disord.* 72, 113-24.

Selye, H., 1975. Stress and distress. *Compr. Ther.* 1, 9-13.

Serradeil-Le Gal, C., Wagnon, J., Simiand, J., Griebel, G., Lacour, C., Guillon, G., Barberis, C., Brossard, G., Soubrie, P., Nisato, D., Pascal, M., Pruss, R., Scatton, B., Maffrand, J.P., Le Fur, G., 2002a. Characterization of (2S,4R)-1-[5-chloro-1-[(2,4-dimethoxyphenyl)sulfonyl]-3-(2-methoxy-phenyl) -2-oxo-2,3-dihydro-1H-indol-3-yl]-4-hydroxy-N,N-dimethyl-2-pyrrolidine carboxamide (SSR149415), a selective and orally active vasopressin V1b receptor antagonist. *J. Pharmacol. Exp. Ther.* 300, 1122-30.

Serradeil-Le Gal, C., Wagnon, J., Valette, G., Garcia, G., Pascal, M., Maffrand, J.P., Le Fur, G., 2002b. Nonpeptide vasopressin receptor antagonists: development of selective and orally active V1a, V2 and V1b receptor ligands. *Prog. Brain Res.* 139, 197-210.

Serradeil-Le Gal, C., Derick, S., Brossard, G., Manning, M., Simiand, J., Gaillard, R., Griebel, G., Guillon, G., 2003. Functional and pharmacological characterization of the first specific agonist and antagonist for the V1b receptor in mammals. *Stress.* 6, 199-206.

Serradeil-Le Gal, C., Wagnon, J., 3rd, Tonnerre, B., Roux, R., Garcia, G., Griebel, G., Aulombard, A., 2005. An overview of SSR149415, a selective nonpeptide vasopressin V(1b) receptor antagonist for the treatment of stress-related disorders. *CNS Drug Rev.* 11, 53-68.

Sharshar, T., Annane, D., 2008. Endocrine effects of vasopressin in critically ill patients. *Best Pract. Res. Clin. Anaesthesiol.* 22, 265-73.

Simonton, O.C., Matthews-Simonton, S., 1981. Cancer and stress: counselling the cancer patient. *Med. J. Aust.* 1, 679, 682-3.

Sokol, H.W., Zimmerman, E.A., 1982. The hormonal status of the Brattleboro rat. *Ann. N Y Acad. Sci.* 394, 535-48.

Sparrenberger, F., Cichelero, F.T., Ascoli, A.M., Fonseca, F.P., Weiss, G., Berwanger, O., Fuchs, S.C., Moreira, L.B., Fuchs, F.D., 2009. Does psychosocial stress cause hypertension? A systematic review of observational studies. *J. Hum. Hypertens.* 23, 12-9.

Spiga, F., Harrison, L.R., MacSweeney, C.P., Thomson, F.J., Craighead, M., Lightman, S.L., 2009a. Effect of vasopressin 1b receptor blockade on the hypothalamic-pituitary-adrenal response of chronically stressed rats to a heterotypic stressor. *J. Endocrinol.* 200, 285-91.

Spiga, F., Harrison, L.R., Wood, S., Knight, D.M., MacSweeney, C.P., Thomson, F., Craighead, M., Lightman, S.L., 2009b. Blockade of the V(1b) receptor reduces ACTH, but not corticosterone secretion induced by stress without affecting basal hypothalamic-pituitary-adrenal axis activity. *J. Endocrinol.* 200, 273-83.

Spirovski, M.Z., Kovacev, V.P., Spasovska, M., Chernick, S.S., 1975. Effect of ACTH on lipolysis in adipose tissue of normal and adrenalectomized rats in vivo. *Am. J. Physiol.* 228, 382-5.

Stark, E., Varga, B., 1968. Effect of ACTH on target-organ blood flow, with special reference to an extra-adrenal effect. *Acta Med. Acad. Sci. Hung.* 25, 367-81.

Stewart, L.Q., Roper, J.A., Young, W.S., 3rd, O'Carroll, A.M., Lolait, S.J., 2008. Pituitary-adrenal response to acute and repeated mild restraint, forced swim and change in environment stress in arginine vasopressin receptor 1b knockout mice. *J. Neuroendocrinol.* 20, 597-605.

Sundaresan, P.R., Guarnaccia, M.M., Izzo, J.L., Jr., 1987. Adrenal medullary regulation of rat renal cortical adrenergic receptors. *Am. J. Physiol.* 253, F1063-7.

Tanoue, A., Ito, S., Honda, K., Oshikawa, S., Kitagawa, Y., Koshimizu, T.A., Mori, T., Tsujimoto, G., 2004. The vasopressin V1b receptor critically regulates hypothalamic-pituitary-adrenal axis activity under both stress and resting conditions. *J. Clin. Invest.* 113, 302-9.

Thorisdottir, S., Johannsson, M., Olafsdottir, E., Arnadottir, M., 2009. Search for the optimal dose interval of adrenocorticotrophic hormone (ACTH(1-24)) with regard to the lipid-lowering effect. *Basic Clin. Pharmacol Toxicol.* 104, 273-5.

Tilders, F.J., Berkenbosch, F., Vermes, I., Linton, E.A., Smelik, P.G., 1985. Role of epinephrine and vasopressin in the control of the pituitary-adrenal response to stress. *Fed. Proc.* 44, 155-60.

Trejter, M., Carraro, G., Rucinski, M., Hochol, A., Rebuffat, P., Nussdorfer, G.G., Malendowicz, L.K., 2005. Arginin-vasopressin regulates proliferative activity of the regenerating rat adrenal cortex. *Int. J. Mol. Med.* 15, 993-7.

Valtin, H., 1982. The discovery of the Brattleboro rat, recommended nomenclature, and the question of proper controls. *Ann. N Y Acad Sci.* 394, 1-9.

van der Meer, M.J., Hermus, A.R., Pesman, G.J., Sweep, C.G., 1996. Effects of cytokines on pituitary beta-endorphin and adrenal corticosterone release in vitro. *Cytokine.* 8, 238-47.

Varga, B., Stark, E., Horvath, E., 1986. Direct effects of ACTH on the ovary. *Acta Physiol. Hung.* 67, 3-11.

Vega, C., Moreno-Carranza, B., Zamorano, M., Quintanar-Stephano, A., Mendez, I., Thebault, S., Martinez de la Escalera, G., Clapp, C., 2010. Prolactin promotes oxytocin and vasopressin release by activating neuronal nitric oxide synthase in the supraoptic and paraventricular nuclei. *Am. J. Physiol. Regul. Integr Comp. Physiol.* 299, R1701-8.

Wotus, C., Osborn, J.W., Nieto, P.A., Engeland, W.C., 2003. Regulation of corticosterone production by vasopressin during water restriction and after drinking in rats. *Neuroendocrinology.* 78, 301-11.

Yasin, S.A., Costa, A., Forsling, M.L., Grossman, A., 1994. Interleukin-1 beta and interleukin-6 stimulate neurohypophysial hormone release in vitro. *J. Neuroendocrinol.* 6, 179-84.

Young, E., Akil, H., 1985. Changes in releasability of ACTH and beta-endorphin with chronic stress. *Neuropeptides.* 5, 545-8.

Zelena, D., Mergl, Z., Foldes, A., Kovacs, K.J., Toth, Z., Makara, G.B., 2003. Role of hypothalamic inputs in maintaining pituitary-adrenal responsiveness in repeated restraint. *Am. J. Physiol. Endocrinol. Metab.* 285, E1110-7.

Zelena, D., Foldes, A., Mergl, Z., Barna, I., Kovacs, K.J., Makara, G.B., 2004. Effects of repeated restraint stress on hypothalamo-pituitary adrenocortical function in vasopressin deficient Brattleboro rats. *Brain Res. Bull.* 63, 521-30.

Zelena, D., Filaretova, L., Mergl, Z., Barna, I., Toth, Z.E., Makara, G.B., 2006a. Hypothalamic paraventricular nucleus, but not vasopressin, participates in chronic hyperactivity of the HPA axis in diabetic rats. *Am. J. Physiol. Endocrinol Metab.* 290, E243-50.

Zelena, D., Mergl, Z., Makara, G.B., 2006b. The role of vasopressin in diabetes mellitus-induced hypothalamo-pituitary-adrenal axis activation: studies in Brattleboro rats. *Brain Res. Bull.* 69, 48-56.

Zelena, D., Barna, I., Csabai, K., Orlando, G.F., Makara, G.B., Engelmann, M., 2008a. Response of the adrenomedullary system to early postnatal stress in the Brattleboro rat. *Ann. N Y Acad. Sci.* 1148, 456-61.

Zelena, D., Domokos, A., Barna, I., Mergl, Z., Haller, J., Makara, G.B., 2008b. Control of the hypothalamo-pituitary-adrenal axis in the neonatal period: adrenocorticotropin and corticosterone stress responses dissociate in vasopressin-deficient brattleboro rats. *Endocrinology.* 149, 2576-83.

Zelena, D., 2009. Yin-Yang Neuropeptides In Depression. *Frontiers in Neuroscience.* 3, 250-251.

Zelena, D., Domokos, A., Jain, S.K., Jankord, R., Filaretova, L., 2009a. The stimuli-specific role of vasopressin in the hypothalamus-pituitary-adrenal axis response to stress. *J. Endocrinol.* 202, 263-78.

Zelena, D., Mergl, Z., Makara, G.B., 2009b. Postnatal development in vasopressin deficient Brattleboro rats with special attention to the hypothalamo-pituitary-adrenal axis function: the role of maternal genotype. *Int. J. Dev. Neurosci.* 27, 175-83.

Zelena, D., Barna, I., Pinter, O., Klausz, B., Varga, J., Makara, G.B., 2011. Congenital absence of vasopressin and age-dependent changes in ACTH and corticosterone stress responses in rats. *Stress.* 14, 420-30.

Zelena, D., Makara, G.B., 2011. *The role of adrenocorticotropin beyond the glucocorticoid horizon in Corticotropin: Pharmacology, Clinical Uses and Adverse Effects,* Nova Pulisher. in press.

Zhou, Y., Leri, F., Cummins, E., Hoeschele, M., Kreek, M.J., 2008. Involvement of arginine vasopressin and V1b receptor in heroin withdrawal and heroin seeking precipitated by stress and by heroin. *Neuropsychopharmacology.* 33, 226-36.

In: Vasopressin
Editor: Leonzio Galella

ISBN: 978-1-62417-311-0

Chapter 2

VASOPRESSIN IN PEDIATRIC SHOCK

Karen Choong
McMaster University, Hamilton, ON, Canada

ABSTRACT

Vasopressin has been used in both adult and pediatric vasodilatory shock and cardiac arrest. The evidence in this area is primarily adult based, while pediatric specific data is more limited. The rationale for vasopressin in shock is based on the following: 1) it reverses the key mechanisms responsible for pathologic vasodilatation and catecholamine resistance, 2) despite its potent systemic vasoconstrictor properties, vasopressin has concurrent organ-specific vasodilator effects that may result in preserved vital organ perfusion; 3) vasopressin influences multiple other hormone responses which may modulate hypothalamic-pituitary axis dysfunction and cellular immune response during septic shock; and 4) vasopressin insufficiency, and an increased sensitivity to the pressor effects of exogenous vasopressin has been demonstrated in both adults and perhaps children with septic shock.

There are to date a total of 40 published pediatric studies evaluating the use of vasopressin in shock, reporting on a collective total of only 642 children. 35 of these studies are in shock, and 5 studies are in cardiac arrest. The vast majority of studies are case reports or case series. Only 2 of these studies are randomized controlled trials (RCT) – one of which was a multi-centred, double-blind RCT of arginine vasopressin in 69 patients vasodilatory shock, while the other was an open-label 58 patient RCT of terlipressin in catecholamine-resistant septic shock While there may be some evidence of short-term benefits with no increased risk of adverse effects, there has been no demonstrable superiority of vasopressin over traditional vasoactive agents on patient important outcomes such as survival, in children with catecholamine-refractory shock and cardio-pulmonary arrest. As a result, vasopressin is not currently recommended as a first line vasoactive agent in pediatric patients with hemodynamic instability. The mortality rate amongst children with shock remains unacceptably high, ranging from 15-70%. As a result, these challenges and controversies rationalize the importance of ongoing prospective research on a potential role for vasopressin in the setting of pediatric shock.

INTRODUCTION

Vasopressin has long been recognized as a potent vasoconstrictor and hence had its primary use in the management of acute gastrointestinal bleeding since the 1950's [1]. However, vasopressin administration in vivo under normal conditions produced only modest increases in systemic blood pressure, and vasopressin antagonists were not shown to be effective anti-hypertensive agents [2]. As a result, it's potential role in the management of shock was not appreciated until 1997 with the emergence of reports of inappropriately low endogenous vasopressin levels, and a hypersensitivity to low-dose exogenous vasopressin in patients with advanced vasodilatory shock [3]. This led to renewed interest and research in this hormone specifically for the management of hemodynamic instability and cardiac arrest. Exogenous vasopressin has now been widely used as a vasopressor in shocked states. Clinical research in this area has been conducted primarily in the adult population, while pediatric specific data is more limited. This chapter will review the physiology of vasopressin, the rationale for its use, and the evidence specifically as it pertains to the management of shock in critically ill children.

PHYSIOLOGY OF VASOPRESSIN DURING SHOCK

Neuroendocrine dysfunction is common during shock and critically illness, and can affect multiple neurohormonal pathways in an individual patient [4]. The hypothalamic-pituitary-adrenal (HPA) axis is a key coordinator of the stress response, and involves a series of complex central and peripheral adaptations essential for survival. The HPA axis is functionally related to the sympathoadrenal system, which is responsible for endogenous catecholamine secretion and inflammatory cytokine activation, as well as the neurohypophyseal system, which is responsible for vasopressin release - all pivotal integrative components in the stress response. Vasopressin is secreted as an adjunct stress hormone to catecholamines in life-threatening situations such as shock and cardiac arrest and therefore plays an important role in homeostasis during cardiovascular instability [5, 6].

Vasopressin Receptor Physiology

Vasopressin is a unique hormone with complex receptor physiology and numerous physiologic functions beyond its vascular actions and osmoregulation [7]. The effects of vasopressin on various vascular beds and tissues are complex. The diversity of its actions are related to the location and density of tissue-specific G-protein-coupled vasopressin receptor subtypes, which are currently classified into V1 vascular, V2 renal, V3 pituitary, oxytocin, and P2 purinergic receptors [8]. Details of each of these individual receptors are further discussed in Chapter). It is now established that vasopressin's vascular actions are primarily mediated through two receptors located in the circulation: V1 receptors (V1-R) and V2 receptors (V2-R) [9]. V1-R vascular receptors are located on vascular smooth muscle and mediate vasoconstriction. However, in the pulmonary circulation, vasopressin activation of V1-R mediates the release of nitric oxide (NO) and causes pulmonary vasodilation, in contrast to its vasoconstrictive action in the systemic circulation. V2-R are located in the collecting duct, where it mediates the hormone's antidiuretic action. V2-R is also expressed in the endothelium, where specific activation of these receptors has been shown to cause vasodilation, and the release of von Willebrand factor. In summary, vasopressin's systemic vasoconstrictor action is primarily mediated through V1-R, while V2-R mediates vasodilation [9, 10].

Regulation of Vasopressin Secretion

The most important stimuli for vasopressin release are increased plasma osmolality, hypotension, and hypovolemia. Under normal conditions, vasopressin plays a minimal role in the vascular regulation of blood pressure, and its main role is in the regulation of water balance [6]. During this time, secretion is regulated primarily by changes in plasma osmolality via input from osmoreceptors, and vasopressin levels may rise as high as 20 pg/mL during maximal urine osmolality [11]. Vasopressin secretion is also under the control of the sympathetic nervous system. Under resting conditions or when stretched, baroreceptors inhibit vasopressin secretion. Decreased activity due to low blood pressure decreases baroreceptor neuronal output and results in the release of vasopressin from the hypothalamus. Non-osmotic stimuli, such as hypovolemia and hypotension, shift the osmotic threshold for vasopressin release to the left, without altering the slope or sensitivity of the relationship of vasopressin and plasma osmolality [12]. Therefore, regardless of plasma osmolality, extremely high levels of vasopressin in the range of 300 –1800 pg/mL, are observed during the initial phase of shock [13]. At these plasma concentrations, vasopressin is a critical mechanism for maintaining systemic vascular resistance and arterial blood pressure, and baroregulation overrides osmoregulation. There is an exponential inverse relationship between plasma vasopressin levels and the degree of hypotension. Small reductions in blood pressure to the order of 5% to 10% from baseline usually have little or no effect on plasma vasopressin, whereas a 20% to 30% decrease results in a 20 to 30-fold increase in serum vasopressin levels [14]. Other important secretagogues of vasopressin include endotoxin and pro-inflammatory cytokines (i.e., interleukin-1β, interleukin-6, tumor necrosis factor-α) [15, 16]. Other non-osmotic stimuli, such as pain, nausea, hypoxia, anesthetic agents, and various endogenous and exogenous chemicals, such as norepinephrine and acetylcholine, may also trigger vasopressin release [17, 18].

Vasopressin Response during Shock

A biphasic vasopressin response has been described in shock, particularly in vasodilatory shock states where high levels are observed in the initial phase of profound hypotension, followed by inappropriately low levels to the order of 3–10 pg/mL, suggesting a depletion in endogenous vasopressin as shock progresses [3, 19, 20]. Several mechanisms responsible for vasopressin deficiency have been proposed, including the depletion of neurohypophyseal stores, impaired baroreflex-mediated release of vasopressin attributable to autonomic dysfunction, and down-regulation of vasopressin production by increased central NO production [11]. The NO-mediated inhibition of vasopressin release may also have important implications in the pathogenesis of adrenal insufficiency, which is commonly observed in critically ill patients, as vasopressin modulates adrenocorticotropic hormone production [21]. It seems unlikely that increased vasopressin clearance from the plasma accounts for vasopressin depletion, given observations that vasopressinase levels remain undetectable in this scenario [22]. Recent studies suggest that cytokines, such as interleukin-1β, tumor necrosis factor-α, and interferon-γ, may also contribute to vasopressin receptor down-regulation and reduced efficacy of exogenous hormone [23].

These observations of endogenous absolute or relative vasopressin deficiency in critically ill adults have been used to justify a role for exogenous vasopressin infusions in patients in refractory shock. Supporting data for absolute or relative vasopressin deficiency from pediatric studies, however, are limited and inconsistent. Several studies have documented low endogenous hormone levels in children with vasodilatory shock prior to starting vasopressin [24-26], however others have reported elevated levels, with no difference between children with septic shock and those without shock [27, 28]. The study by Mastropietro et al suggests that plasma vasopressin stores are depleted in a subset of children following cardiopulmonary bypass, however this does not reliably identify which patients are more likely to develop a low cardiac output state. Patients with the combination of hemodynamic instability and low vasopressin levels did however have a demonstrable hemodynamic improvement following the administration of exogenous vasopressin [29].

There are several possible explanations for the inconsistencies in vasopressin levels between adult and pediatric patients. Children with septic shock present with different hemodynamic physiology than their adult counterparts [30]. Low cardiac index, high systemic vascular resistance shock is more common than vasodilatory shock in children, and this hemodynamic status often changes over time [31]. The observations in adults clearly identify endogenous vasopressin deficiency, especially in vasodilatory shock, while the pediatric studies are inconsistent in that both cold and warm shock patients were not distinguished. These clinical differences between children and adults with shock reflect the age-related complexity of pathophysiologic mechanisms, which extends beyond vasopressin dysregulation. There are also limitations in the measurement of plasma vasopressin. Therefore, the reliability of endogenous vasopressin levels as a marker for its use and likelihood of a positive hemodynamic response to exogenous vasopressin infusions has not been adequately explored in children.

Assessing the Vasopressin Axis During Shock

As a result of these reports of inappropriately low vasopressin levels during shock, identifying vasopressin deficient individuals may guide management and prognosis. However, the detection of endogenous deficiency by measuring circulating vasopressin levels is limited by the fact that the mature hormone is unstable, has a short half-life, and circulates largely attached to platelets. Hence, interpretation of static measurements of vasopressin may be misleading. Copeptin, a stable vasopressin precursor, is secreted in an equimolar ratio and thus mirrors the production of vasopressin [32]. Copeptin is a more stable surrogate marker for vasopressin release, and has therefore been proposed as a more sensitive and potential prognostic biomarker in sepsis [33, 34]. Others have suggested that the ratio of vasopressin to norepinephrine levels should be considered a reflection of adequacy of vasopressin homeostasis relative to adrenocorticoid homeostasis. The vasopressin/norepinephrine ratios in sepsis and severe sepsis are similar (1/175) while they are much lower when shock ensues (1/1000) [35].

The Role of Vasopressin in the Management of Shock

Vasopressin has been used in both adult and pediatric cardiac arrest as well as vasodilatory shock states from a variety of underlying causes such as septic shock, post-perfusion syndrome following cardio-pulmonary bypass, prolonged hemorrhage, and in hemodynamically unstable organ donors [36-40]. Although vasodilatory shock may result from multiple different causes, there are common pathogenic mechanisms that result in vascular smooth muscle dysfunction and vascular hyporesponsiveness to catecholamines [41]. Three mechanisms have been implicated: activation of the adenosine triphosphate (ATP)-sensitive and calcium-regulated potassium channels in the plasma membrane of vascular smooth muscle, activation of the inducible form of nitric oxide synthase, and depletion of the pituitary stores of vasopressin [42].

Vasoconstrictor Effects of Vasopressin

Vasopressin directly inactivates in vascular smooth muscle, a critical mechanism responsible for the pathologic vasodilation and resistance to catecholamine pressors that characterize vasodilatory shock. In addition, vasopressin blunts the increase in cyclic guanosine monophosphate induced by NO and atrio-natriuretic peptide and inhibits the production of interleukin-1β, mechanisms strongly implicated in the pathogenesis of vasodilation [43]. While inappropriately low plasma vasopressin levels have been described in adults and pediatric patients with vasodilatory shock, such patients appear to demonstrate a hypersensitivity to the pressor effects of exogenous vasopressin [3, 11, 39]. The overall effect of vasopressin on systemic blood pressure is minimal at normal plasma concentrations and in healthy individuals (8, 44). Although vasopressin infusions of 0.2–2 units/min rarely affect blood pressure in euvolemic or normotensive subjects, low-dose infusions of 0.04 units/min substantially increase systemic pressure in patients with catecholamine-refractory hypotension. It is likely that because plasma vasopressin is low in this condition, its vascular receptors are available for occupancy by exogenous hormone. In contrast, exogenous norepinephrine may not increase receptor occupancy to the same extent, as endogenous concentrations of norepinephrine are high, which in turn may cause desensitization of receptors [44]. Furthermore, there is evidence for adrenergic receptor down-regulation in addition to hyperpolarization from the activation of ATP-sensitive potassium channels, which results in decreased vascular sensitivity to catecholamines despite high endogenous concentrations and exogenous infusions. The administration of low-dose vasopressin, however, has been shown to not only initiate vasoconstriction but also potentiate the vasoconstrictor effects of catecholamine pressors [45].

Vasodilator Effects of Vasopressin

Although vasopressin is a potent systemic vasoconstrictor, the same low-dose infusion of vasopressin concurrently causes vasodilation in pulmonary, cerebral, and coronary circulations via oxytocin receptor stimulation and endothelial NO release [8]. Low-dose vasopressin may thus be more beneficial in preserving vital organ perfusion when compared with catecholamine pressors. Investigators have demonstrated in patients with septic shock that low-dose vasopressin not only improved mean arterial blood pressure and cerebral perfusion pressure but also spared the microcirculation to the mesenteric and renal beds when compared with norepinephrine or phenylephrine [46, 47].

Renovascular Effects

Paradoxically, vasopressin (also known as antidiuretic hormone) can increase urine output and creatinine clearance in patients with septic shock when compared with norepinephrine [48, 49]. This effect has been attributed to V1-R mediated, selective renal efferent arteriolar constriction. In contrast, increasing doses of catecholamine vasopressor agents increase the resistance in both afferent and efferent glomerular arterioles, which can contribute to decreased glomerular filtration rate and creatinine clearance and thus decreased urine output.

Endocrine Effects

Vasopressin is a potent stimulator of adrenocorticotropic hormone and, consequently, cortisol release [50], which are important considerations given the prevalence of adrenocortical dysfunction in the critically ill population [51]. The interaction of corticotropin and vasopressin release in shock is complex and incompletely understood, and the influence of exogenous administrations of vasopressin and steroids on the respective axes is being explored. Since corticosteroids have been shown to reverse tachyphylaxis against exogenous catecholamines, it has been suggested through an ovine model of endotoxemia that methylprednisolone may reverse vasopressin hyporesponsiveness [23]. Vasopressin has also been reported to mediate atrial natriuretic factor and angiotensin II secretion as well as stimulate prolactin and endothelin I release [52]. This latter effect on prolactin secretion plays a significant role in the cellular immune response, which in turn has important implications in the critically ill population with septic shock.

In summary, vasopressin is a an attractive adjunctive agent in the management of shock and cardiac arrest for the following reasons:

1) It reverses the key mechanisms responsible for pathologic vasodilatation and catecholamine resistance observed in vasodilatory and refractory shock [41]; 2) despite its potent systemic

vasoconstrictor properties, vasopressin has concurrent organ-specific vasodilator effects that may result in preserved vital organ perfusion; 3) vasopressin influences multiple other hormone responses which may modulate HPA axis dysfunction and cellular immune response during septic shock [43, 49, 52]; and 4) vasopressin insufficiency, and an increased sensitivity to the pressor effects of exogenous vasopressin has been demonstrated in both adults and perhaps children with septic shock [53].

VASOPRESSIN PHARMACOLOGY IN SHOCK

The most commonly used and extensively researched forms of vasopressin in the setting of shock are arginine vasopressin (AVP) and terlipressin.

Arginine Vasopressin

While its primary action is mediated through V1 and V2 receptors, AVP may also act on the oxytocin receptors at high concentrations. AVP is not protein-bound, and has a volume of distribution of 140 L/kg. The plasma half-life of AVP is approximately 24 minutes which lends itself to administration by continuous infusion during the management of vasodilatory shock [35]. Approximately 65% is cleared by renal elimination, with the remaining approximately 35% is metabolized by tissue peptidases. Given it's short half-life AVP is typically administered as a continuous infusion in the setting of shock. The reported effective dose ranges used in pediatric shock have been variable, and are outlined in Tables 1 and 2.

Terlipressin

Terlipressin (tri-glycyl lysine vasopressin) is a synthetic analogue of lysine vasopressin. Terlipressin behaves as a pro-drug, and is converted to lysine vasopressin in the circulation after the N-trigylcyl residue is cleaved by endothelial peptidases. Terlipressin has a similar pharmacodynamic profile but a much longer effective half-life than AVP of approximately 6 hours. The elimination half-life is around 50 minutes [54]. Terlipressin is typically administered as an intravenous bolus in children (10-20 mcg/kg), however it has been used as an infusion [55-57].

There has been some recent experimental animal data suggesting that selective V2-R antagonism may be an innovative approach to maintaining end-organ perfusion in early septic shock [58]. This has yet to be evaluated in human studies.

Which is the Most Effective Vasopressin?

AVP exerts its principal effect via V1a receptor stimulation, however its action on V2 receptors may exacerbate undesireable adverse effects in septic shock such as hypercoagulation, antidiuresis, selective vasodilation, and CNS changes [59, 60]. Terlipressin is believed to have higher selectivity for the V1 receptor than AVP (V1/V2 ratio 2.2 vs 1), and may be more potent in reversing vasodilation in the setting of vasodilatory shock. The potential downside of its action is the risk of excessive systemic and pulmonary vascular resistance, and micro-regional vasoconstriction after bolus injection, which may be avoided with continuous low dose terlipressin infusions [61]. Continuous low-dose terlipressin infusion (1.3 mcg/kg/h) has been compared to AVP (0.03 U/min) and shown to reduce on open-label norepinephrine requirements in septic shock adults [55]. However, there are no studies in either the adult or pediatric literature suggesting the superiority of one form of vasopressin to the other.

Vasopressin Therapy in Shock – The Evidence

Exogenous vasopressin and its analogues have most commonly be used and researched in the setting of cardiac arrest and a variety of vasodilatory shock states. Most of the research is from the adult literature. We will first summarize the findings from adult trials, followed by the pediatric specific literature.

Evidence in Adults

There are at least 8 randomized controlled trials and numerous observational studies on AVP or terlipressin in the management of vasodilatory shock in adults. The majority of these trials were in vasodilatory septic shock, and compared AVP or terlipressin to norepinephrine. In these 10 trials, the primary outcome was mean arterial pressure (4 trials) [11, 62-64], norepinephrine or catecholamine requirements (3 trials) [48, 55, 65], and 28-day mortality (1 trial) [66]. The Vasopressin and Septic Shock Trial (VASST) conducted by Russell et al. is the largest of the adult trials [66]. VASST evaluated the effect of low dose AVP (0.01-0.03 U/min) as an adjunctive agent compared to norepinephrine alone, on mortality in 779 adult patients in septic shock [67]. There was no difference in 28-day mortality between groups (35.4% vs. 39.3%, $P = 0.26$). Although the authors had predicted that based on its vasoconstrictor potency, AVP would be more efficacious in the stratum of patients with more severe septic shock (baseline requirement of ≥ 15 µg/kg/min norepinephrine), they observed a significant reduction in mortality in the subgroup of patients with less severe septic shock (baseline of 5-14 µg/kg/min norepinephrine). While the authors conclude that these subgroup findings should be hypothesis generating only, it has sparked further debate as to whether higher doses of vasopressin should be used in patients with more severe shock, and should be thus evaluated in future studies. A meta-analysis of trials conducted by the European Society of Intensive Care Medicine (ESICM) Systematic Review Group published in 2012 revealed that the use of AVP or terlipressin did not result in a short term survival benefit in patients with vasodilatory shock (RR 0.91; 95% CI 0.79 – 1.05) [68]. There was no increased risk of serious adverse events from AVP or terlipressin therapy. Treatment with vasopressin did significantly reduce norepinephrine requirements, and therefore the authors concluded that physicians may value the norepinephrine sparing effect of vasopressin given its apparent safe profile.

Potential interaction between vasopressin and corticosteroids has led to the suggestion that the combination of 2 hormones may be beneficial in the management of septic shock through the following mechanisms: vasopressin increases ACTH secretion by corticotropic cells through V1b receptors during stress [69]; corticosteroids and vasopressin both block ATP-sensitive potassium channels, the activation of which results in abnormal vasodilation [70, 71]; corticosteroids may also increase the sensitivity of V1a-receptors, which are suspected to be down-regulated in sepsis [72]. A post hoc analysis of the VASST trial suggested that combined vasopressin and corticosteroid therapy was associated with decreased mortality and organ dysfunction than norepinephrine and corticosteroids [73]. A subsequent open-label trial by Torgersen and colleagues demonstrated that higher doses of AVP (0.067 IU/min) resulted in improved hemodynamic control without increased adverse effects, compared to lower doses of 0.033 IU/min in patients with vasodilatory septic shock [74]. Pooled results from studies of vasopressin in addition to corticosteroids have failed to demonstrate a mortality benefit in adults with septic shock [75]. The combination of corticosteroids and vasopressin has not been systematically evaluated in children to date, however in the randomized controlled trial of AVP in pediatric shock by Choong et al, there was no difference in outcomes in the subgroup of patients who received corticosteroids [24]. In summary, there is insufficient evidence at present supporting the use of vasopressin either alone or in combination with corticosteroids, in the setting of vasodilatory or septic shock.

Experimental protocols for cardiopulmonary resuscitation (CPR) in adults and animals have suggested that vasopressin is superior to epinephrine in increasing vital organ blood flow, in particular coronary arterial and cerebral blood flow, when administered intravenously as well as endobronchially or via intraosseous route [76]. In a prospective study of 40 patients with out-of- hospital ventricular fibrillation resistant to electrical defibrillation, a significantly larger number of patients who received 40 units of vasopressin intravenously compared with 1 mg of epinephrine were successfully resuscitated and survived for 24 hrs [77]. However, an in-hospital cardiac arrest, triple-blind, randomized controlled trial failed to demonstrated a survival advantage for vasopressin over epinephrine [78]. Subsequently, a comparison of vasopressin and epinephrine for out-of-hospital cardiac arrest, which included 1,186 adult patients, demonstrated a significantly better outcome among patients with asystole who received vasopressin, although no significant difference in outcome was demonstrated in patients with ventricular tachycardia or pulseless electrical activity [79].

A systematic review and meta-analysis of 5 randomized controlled trials of vasopressin compared to epinephrine in adult patients wit cardiac arrest revealed that there was no statistically significant differences between the 2 groups in return of spontaneous circulation, death before hospital admission, within 24 hours, of before hospital discharge, or composite outcome of death or neurologically impaired survivors.

Subgroup analyses also showed no statistical difference in these outcomes depending on the cardiac rhythm at presentation (ventricular fibrillation or tachycardia, pulseless electrical activity of asystole) [80]. In summary, current evidence does not demonstrate any clear advantage of vasopressin over epinephrine in the treatment of cardiac arrest in adults.

Evidence in Pediatrics

Inspired by concurrent research in the adult population, researchers began to evaluate the efficacy of vasopressin in shock in the pediatric population. Our review of Medline and Embase from 1966 to August 2012 revealed a total of 40 published pediatric studies evaluating the use of AVP or terlipressin, reporting on a collective total of only 642 children, since the first reports of its use in pediatric shock in 1999 [25] 35 of these studies are in shock, while 5 studies are in cardiac arrest. The vast majority of studies are case reports or case series. The doses used in these studies varied substantively, ranging from 0.00002 U/kg/min to 0.003 U/kg/min of AVP, and terlipressin dosing administered in the range of 10-20 mcg/kg anywhere from every 4 to 12 hourly, to continuous infusion (10-20mcg/kg/h) [53, 81]. Many of the observational studies suggested that AVP or terlipressin decreased traditional vasoactive infusion requirements, and increases urine output in children with catecholamine-resistant shock [53, 82]. The overall mortality rate in this study population is high (43.9%), despite the use of vasopressin [83]. However, none of these studies were designed nor adequately powered for mortality as an outcome, which is a major limitation in pediatric critical care research.

Table 1. Prospective and comparative studies of Vasopressin in pediatric shock

Reference	Study Design	Clinical Setting	Dose	Sample size	Main Findings	Adverse Events
Arginine Vasopressin (AVP)						
Alten, 2012[95]	Retrospective case-control	Neonates following complex cardiac surgery	0.0003 U/kg/min	19 AVP, 18 controls	Decreased fluid resuscitation and catecholamine requirements in 1st 24h post-operative, and earlier net negative fluid balance with AVP	Lower serum sodium in first 48 hours with AVP (132 vs. 137 mmol/L, p=0.01)
Agrawal, 2012[96]	Prospective cohort	Post cardiac surgery, catecholamine refractory vasodilatory shock	0.0005 – 0.003 U//kg/min	12	Improvement in MAP, inotropic requirement and serum lactate from baseline.	3 deaths, one death while on AVP. Drop in platelet count while on AVP.

Table 1. (Continued)

Reference	Study Design	Clinical Setting	Dose	Sample size	Main Findings	Adverse Events
Choong, 2009[24]	Multi-centre, double blind, RCT	Vasodilatory Shock	0.0005-0.002 U/kg/min	69	No significant difference in vasoactive-free hemodynamic stability, organ failure free days, length of stay and mortality	Trend towards increased mortality with AVP (30% vs 15.6%, RR 1.94, 95% CI 0.75-5.05; p=0.24). No significant difference in digital ischemia, thrombocytopenia, and arrhythmias.
Meyer, 2006[97]	Prospective cohort	Very low-birthweight infants with catecholamine resistant septic and cardiogenic shock	0.01 – 0.1 U/kg/h	3	Transient improvement in MAP	2 deaths
Katz, 2000[38]	Retrospective case-control	Critically ill children during brain death and organ recovery	0.041+/-0.069 U/kg/h	34 AVP, 29 controls	Significantly higher MAP, and ability to wean off catecholamines with AVP.	No adverse effect on organ recovery function. No reported AVP induced dysrhythmia, hypertension, anuria or toxicity.
Terlipressin (TP)						
Yildizdas, 2008[84]	Single centre, open-lable RCT	Catecholamine refractory septic shock	20 mcg/kg Q 6h for a maximum of 96h	58	Significant increased in MAP and PaO2/FiO2 ratio. No significant difference in mortality (67.3% vs 71.4%)	No reported difference in adverse events
Rodriguez-Nunez, 2006[98]	Prospective cohort	Catecholamine refractory septic shock	0.2 mg/kg Q4 h	16	Rapid improvement in MAP, reduction in catecholamines in 14/16 patients	9 deaths. 9 ischemic sequelae, 5 possibly related to TP. 1 oliguria, 2 rhabdomyolysis, 1 hyperkalemia, and 1 hyperbilirubinemia

MAP, mean arterial pressure; RR, relative risk; CI, confidence interval.

Vasopressin has most commonly been studied in the setting of catecholamine-resistant or vasodilatory shock in children, either secondary to sepsis or post-cardiopulmonary bypass. There are only 5 prospective studies, and one retrospective case-control study, which are summarized in Table 1. Only 2 of these studies are randomized controlled trials (RCT) – one of which was a multi-centred, double-blind RCT of vasopressin in 69 patients vasodilatory shock [24], while the other was an open-label 58 patient RCT of terlipressin in catecholamine-resistant septic shock [84]. The Vasopressin in Pediatric Vasodilatory Shock trial which evaluated the safety and efficacy of low dose vasopressin as an adjunctive agent found no difference in the time to hemodynamic stability, organ free failure days and magnitude of vasoactive agent use and between the vasopressin and placebo groups [24]. While there was no difference in the adverse event rates, there was a non-statistically significant trend towards increased mortality in the vasopressin group (30.3% vs 15.6%; p = 0.24). The trial by Yildizdas et al found that terlipressin increased systemic blood pressure, however, this did not lead to a significant mortality benefit (67.3% vs. 71.4%) [84].

In pediatric asphyxial animal models, vasopressin alone during CPR was less effective than epinephrine alone, whereas vasopressin plus epinephrine was as effective as epinephrine alone [85]. However, when cardiac arrest was evoked by ventricular fibrillation, the combination of vasopressin and epinephrine was superior to either drug alone for resuscitation [86]. There are only a total of 5 published reports of AVP or terlipressin use in pediatric cardio-pulmonary arrest (Table 2). All of these studies are retrospective reviews. All studies evaluated the use of vasopressin in pediatric in-patients receiving CPR, who were unresponsive to conventional therapy (epinephrine and or cardioversion). The largest series of these studies is from the American Heart Association National Registry of pediatric resuscitation, reporting on a total of 1293 consecutive pediatric patients with pulseless cardiac arrest in 176 North American Hospitals between October 1999 to November 2004 [87]. Only 5% of pediatric patients received vasopressin during cardiac arrest in this review. Vasopressin was most often given in a pediatric hospital (57%) and in and intensive care setting (76.6%). Return of spontaneous circulation occurred in 32 of 71 (45%) patients, and survival to hospital discharge was 14%. Patients who were given vasopressin had longer arrest duration (median 37 minutes) vs. those who did not (24 minutes) (p = 0.004). In multivariate analysis, vasopressin was associated with worse ROSC but no difference in 24 hours or discharge survival.

Table 2. Vasopressin in Pediatric Cardiac Arrest Studies

Reference	Study Design	Setting	Drug and Dosage	n	Main Findings
Yildizdas, 2011[94]	Retrospective case series	In-hospital cardiac arrests unresponsive to conventional therapy	Terlipressin, 20 mcg/kg, range of 1-4 doses	12 events in 9 patients	ROSC in 6 of 12 episodes. 5 survivors, no significant neurological sequelae
Gil-Anton, 2010[99]	Multi-centre registry	In-PICU cardiac arrest unresponsive to at least 3 epinephrine doses	Teripressin 10-20 mcg/kg up to 2 doses	5 patients	Sustained ROSC in 4 patients. 2 survivors, no significant neurological sequelae.
Matok, 2007[40]	Retrospective case series	All PCCU patients treated with terlipressin during CPR	Terlipressin; 15-20 mcg/kg/dose	7 patients	ROSC in 6 of 8 episodes; 4 survivors to discharge with no neurologic sequelae.
Duncan, 2009[87]	Multi-centred, National Registry	In-hospital CPR	Vasopressin	1293 patients	5% of patients received vasopressin. Vasopressin was associated with longer arrest duration, worse ROSC and no difference in 24 h and discharge survival
Mann, 2002[100]	Retrospective case series	In-hospital pediatric cardiac arrests unresponsive to conventional therapy	Vasopressin, 0.4 U/kg/dose	4 patients	ROSC in 3 of 4 patients; 1 survival to hospital discharge

ROSC, return of spontaneous circulation; PCCU pediatric critical care unit; CPR, cardiopulmonary resuscitation.

In light of the current evidence, vasopressin is recognized as a potential alternative vasopressor when standard therapies fail to restore spontaneous circulation. However, no firm recommendations exist concerning the use of vasopressin for CPR in infants and children, and more prospective clinical trial evidence is clearly needed.

Safety of Vasopressin in Pediatric Shock

Because of its potent vasoconstrictor action, potential adverse effects of low dose vasopressin include increase in myocardial after-load, reductions in oxygen delivery, impaired tissues perfusion and ischemic tissue injury. Thrombocytopenia and increases in aminotransferases activity and bilirubin concentrations have also been reported. These adverse effects appear to be dose-dependent, and more commonly noted with doses of greater than 0.04 U/min of vasopressin or 2 μg/kg/h of terlipressin [35]. However, some of the data is conflicting, and it is yet unclear whether the hemodynamic alterations represent adaptive response to stabilized blood pressure, or the impaired tissue perfusion is an epiphenomenon of the severity of underlying disease rather than a specific side effect of vasopressin or concurrent catecholamine pressor administration [88]. The largest of the adult and pediatric clinical trials, VASST and Vasopressin in Pediatric Vasodilatory Shock trial, reported no significant difference in adverse event rates between the vasopressin and control groups [67, 89].

CONCLUSION

Current evidence with respect to vasopressin use in pediatric shock are based on a handful of adequately conducted trials, which are significantly fewer in number and underpowered when compared to adult literature. Regardless, the conclusions from prospective trials to date are similar. While there may be some indication of short-term benefits with no increased risk of adverse effects, there has been no demonstrable superiority of vasopressin over traditional vasoactive agents on patient important outcomes such as survival, in patients with catecholamine-refractory or vasodilatory shock, or following cardiopulmonary arrest. As a result, vasopressin is not currently recommended as the first line vasoactive agent of choice in adults and pediatric patients with hemodynamic instability [90]. Based on the results of VASST, low dose vasopressin infusion may be considered as an adjunctive agent, however, with the anticipation of an effect equivalent to that of norepinephrine alone in adults. However, there is no evidence that adjunctive vasopressin therapy is beneficial in pediatric shock at the present time. There are currently no recommendations for routine testing for endogenous vasopressin levels in the setting of shock in light of the challenges and its lack of utility in indicating potential responders. However, its precursor copeptin, may prove to be a more sensitive and prognostic biomarker in sepsis.

Numerous controversies remain with respect to vasopressin in the management of shock, which fuel ongoing interest in this hormone. These include the following: 1) appropriate patient selection – identifying the patient physiology that may most benefit from vasopressin such as vasodilatory shock; 2) timing of the intervention (early versus rescue therapy); 3) appropriate dosage – is there a dose response on efficacy as well as safety; and 4) the most appropriate outcomes particularly in pediatrics, given that systemic blood pressure is not a good surrogate for organ function and survival. These factors are not unique to the study of vasopressin, and hence despite decades of research, it is difficult to identify a single superior vasoactive agent for the management of shock [91, 92]. Furthermore, the management of shock in pediatrics has added challenges given the broad age range from preterm neonates to adolescence, its heterogeneous presentation, and the limitations with the clinical assessment of hemodynamic physiology in children [93]. Vasoactive therapy should ideally be tailored and titrated according to the patient's physiological and clinical status. As with any vasoactive therapy, close monitoring of end-organ perfusion, awareness of potential side effects, and the measurement of tissue flow where possible are essential. The mortality rate amongst children with shock remains unacceptably high, ranging from 15-70% [24, 94]. As a result, these challenges and controversies rationalize the importance of ongoing prospective research on a potential role for vasopressin in the setting of pediatric shock.

REFERENCES

[1] Tuggle DW, Bennett KG, Scott J, Tunell WP. Intravenous vasopressin and gastrointestinal hemorrhage in children. *J Pediatr Surg.* 1988 Jul;23(7):627-9.

[2] Landry D, Oliver J. Increased complexity of vasopressin's vascular actions. *Crit Care.* 2010;14:1011.

[3] Landry DW, Levin HR, Gallant EM, Ashton RC, Seo S, D'Alessandro D, et al. Vasopressin deficiency contributes to the vasodilation of septic shock. *Circulation.* 1997 Mar 4;95(5):1122-5.

[4] Hebbar K, Rigby M, Felner E, Easley K, Fortenberry J. Neuroendocrine dysfunction in pediatric critical illness. *Pediatr Crit Care Med.* 2009;10:35-40.

[5] Treshcan T, Peters J. The vasopressin system: Physiology and clinical stategies. *Anesthesiology.* 2006;105:599-612.

[6] Forrest P. Vasopressin and Shock. *Anaesth Intensive Care.* 2001;29:463-72.

[7] Treshcan T, Peters J. The vasopressin sys-tem: Physiology and clinical strategies. *Anesthesiology.* 2006;105:599-612.

[8] Holmes CL, Landry DW, Granton JT. Science review: Vasopressin and the cardiovascular system part 1-receptor physiology. *Crit Care.* 2003 Dec;7(6):427-34.

[9] Maybauer M, Maybauer D, Enkhbaatar P, Traber D. Physiology of the vasopressin receptors. *Best Practice and Research.* 2008;22(2):253-63.

[10] Bichet DG, Razi M, Lonergan M, Arthus MF, Papukna V, Kortas C, et al. Hemodynamic and coagulation responses to 1-desamino[8-D-arginine] vasopressin in patients with congenital nephrogenic diabetes insipidus. *N Engl J Med.* 1988 Apr 7;318(14):881-7.

[11] Dunser M, Wenzel V, Mayr A, Hasibeder W. Management of vasodilatory shock: defining the role of arginine vasopressin. *Drugs.* 2003;63(3):237-56.

[12] Shrier R, Bert T, Anderson R. Osomotic and nonosmotic control of vasopressin release. *Am J Physiol.* 1979;236:F321-F32.

[13] Oliver J, Landry D. Endogenous and exogenous vasopressin in shock. *Curr Opin Crit Care.* 2007;13(4):376-82.

[14] Hirsch A, Majzoub J, Ren C, Scales K, Creager M. Contribution of vasopressin to blood pressure regulation during hypovolemic hypotension in humans. *Journal of Applied Physiology.* 1993;75(5):1984-8.

[15] Kasting N, Mazurek K, Martin J. Endotoxin increases vasopressin release independently of known physiologic stimuli. *Am J Physiol.* 1985;238(4):E420-E4.

[16] Chikanza I, Petrou P, Chrousos G. Perturbations of arginine vasopressin secretion during inflammatory stress: Pathophysiologic implications. *Ann NY Acad Sci.* 2000;917(1):825-34.

[17] Gerigk K, Gnehm H, Rascher W. Arginine vasopressin and renin in acutely ill children: implication for fluid therapy. *Acta Paediatr.* 1996;85(5):550-3.

[18] Neville K, Verge C, M OM, Walker J. HIgh antidiuretic hormone levels and hyponatremia in children with gastroenteritis. *Pediatrics.* 2005;116(6):1401-7.

[19] Sharshar T, Blanchard A, Paillard M, Raphael J, Gajdos P, Annane D. Circulating vasopresin levels in septic shock. *Crit Care Med.* 2003;31(6):1752-8.

[20] Tsuneyoshi I, Yamada H, Kakihana Y, Nakamura M, Nakano Y, Boyle WA, 3rd. Hemodynamic and metabolic effects of low-dose vasopressin infusions in vasodilatory septic shock. *Crit Care Med.* 2001 Mar;29(3):487-93.

[21] Robin JK, Oliver JA, Landry DW. Vasopressin deficiency in the syndrome of irreversible shock. *J Trauma.* 2003 May;54(5 Suppl):S149-54.
[22] Sharshar T, Carlier R, Balnchard A, Feydy A, Gray F, Paillard M, et al. Depletion of neurophyseal content of vasopressin in septic shock. *Crit Care Med.* 2002;30(3):497-500.
[23] Ertmer C, Bone H-G, Morelli A, Van Aken H, Erren M, Lange M, et al. Methylprednisolone reverses vasopressin hyporesponsiveness in ovine endotoxemia. *Shock.* 2007;27(3):281-8.
[24] Choong K, Bohn D, Fraser D, Gaboury I, Hutchison J, Joffe A, et al. Vasopressin in Pediatric Vasodilatory Shock. A Muticentre Randomized Controlled Trial. *Am J Respir Crit Care Med.* 2009;180:632-9.
[25] Rosenzweig EB, Starc TJ, Chen JM, Cullinane S, Timchak DM, Gersony WM, et al. Intravenous arginine-vasopressin in children with vasodilatory shock after cardiac surgery. *Circulation.* 1999 Nov 9;100(19 Suppl):II182-6.
[26] Masutani S, Senzaki H, Ishido H, Taketazu M, Matsunaga T, Kobayashi T, et al. Vasopressin in the treatment of vasodilatory shock in children. *Pediatr Int.* 2005;47(2):132-6.
[27] Lodha R, Vivekanandhan S, Sarthi M, Kabra S. Serial circulating vasopressin levels in children with septic shock. *Pediatr Crit Care Med.* 2006;7(3):220-4.
[28] Leclerc F, Walter-Nicolet E, Leteurtre S, Noizet O, Sadik A, Cremer R, et al. Admission plasma vasopressin levels in children with meningococcal septic shock. *Intensive Care Med.* 2003 Aug;29(8):1339-44.
[29] Mastropietro C, Rossi N, Clark J, Chen H, Walters 3rd H, Delius R, et al. Relative deficiency of arginine vasopressin in children after cardiopulmonary bypass. *Crit Care Med.* 2010;38(10):2052-8.
[30] Carcillo JA, Pollack MM, Ruttimann UE, Fields AI. Sequential physiologic interactions in pediatric cardiogenic and septic shock. *Crit Care Med.* 1989 Jan;17(1):12-6.
[31] Ceneviva G, Paschall JA, Maffei F, Carcillo JA. Hemodynamic support in fluid-refractory pediatric septic shock. *Pediatrics.* 1998 Aug;102(2):e19.
[32] Müller B, Morgenthaler N, Stolz D, Schuetz P, Müller C, Bingisser R, et al. Circulating levels of copeptin, a novel biomarker, in lower respiratory tract infections. *Eur J clin invest.* 2007;37(2):145-52.

[33] Morgenthaler N, Struck J, Jochberger S, Dunser M. Copeptin: clinical use of a new biomarker. *Trends in Endocrinology and Metabolism.* 2008;19(2):43-9.

[34] Nickel C, Bingisser R, Morgenthaler N. The role of copeptin as a diagnostic and prognostic biomarker for risk stratification in the emergency department. *BMC Medicine.* 2012;10(7):doi:10.1186/741-7015-10-7.

[35] Russell J. Vasopressin in vasodilatory and septic shock. *Current Opinion in Critical Care.* 2007;13:383-91.

[36] Argenziano M, Choudhri AF, Oz MC, Rose EA, Smith CR, Landry DW. A prospective randomized trial of arginine vasopressin in the treatment of vasodilatory shock after left ventricular assist device placement. *Circulation.* 1997 Nov 4;96(9 Suppl):II-286-90.

[37] Dunser MW, Mayr AJ, Ulmer H, Knotzer H, Sumann G, Pajk W, et al. Arginine vasopressin in advanced vasodilatory shock: a prospective, randomized, controlled study. *Circulation.* 2003 May 13;107(18):2313-9.

[38] Katz K, Lawler J, Wax J, O'Connor R, Nadkarni V. Vasopressin pressor effects in critically ill children during evaluation for brain death and organ recovery. *Resuscitation.* 2000;47(1):33-40.

[39] Mastropietro C, Davalos M, Seshadri S, Walters H, Delius R. Clinical response to arginine vasopressin therapy after paediatric cardiac surgery. *Cardiol Young.* 2012:1-7 [Epub ahead of print].

[40] Matok I, Vardi A, Augarten A, Efrati O, Leibovitch L, Rubinshtein M, et al. Beneficial effects of terlipressin in prolonged pediatric cardiopulmonary resuscitation: a case series. *Critical care medicine.* [Case Reports]. 2007 Apr;35(4):1161-4.

[41] Landry DW, Oliver JA. The pathogenesis of vasodilatory shock. *N Engl J Med.* 2001 Aug 23;345(8):588-95.

[42] Holmes C, Walley K. Arginine vasopressin in the treatment of vasodilatory shock. *Best Practice and Research Clinical Anaesthesiology.* 2008;22(2):275-86.

[43] Holmes CL, Landry DW, Granton JT. Science Review: Vasopressin and the cardiovascular system part 2 - clinical physiology. *Crit Care.* 2004 Feb;8(1):15-23.

[44] Thiemermann C, Szabo C, Mitchell JA, Vane JR. Vascular hyporeactivity to vasoconstrictor agents and hemodynamic decompensation in hemorrhagic shock is mediated by nitric oxide. *Proc Natl Acad Sci U S A.* 1993 Jan 1;90(1):267-71.

[45] Bartelstone HJ, Nasmyth PA. Vasopressin Potentiation of Catecholamine Actions in Dog, Rat, Cat, and Rat Aortic Strip. *Am J Physiol.* 1965 Apr;208:754-62.

[46] Dubois MJ, De Backer D, Creteur J, Anane S, Vincent JL. Effect of vasopressin on sublingual microcirculation in a patient with distributive shock. *Intensive Care Med.* 2003 Jun;29(6):1020-3.

[47] Malay MB, Ashton JL, Dahl K, Savage EB, Burchell SA, Ashton RC, Jr., et al. Heterogeneity of the vasoconstrictor effect of vasopressin in septic shock. *Crit Care Med.* 2004 Jun;32(6):1327-31.

[48] Patel BM, Chittock DR, Russell JA, Walley KR. Beneficial effects of short-term vasopressin infusion during severe septic shock. *Anesthesiology.* 2002 Mar;96(3):576-82.

[49] Holmes CL, Landry DW, Granton JT. Science review: Vasopressin and the cardiovascular system part 1--receptor physiology. *Crit Care.* 2003;7(6):427-34.

[50] Bilezikjian L, Vale W. Regulation of ACTH secretion from corticotrophs: The interaction of vasopressin and CRF. *Ann NY Acad Sci.* 1987;512:85-96.

[51] Annane D. Corticosteroids for septic shock. *Crit Care Med.* 2001 Jul;29(7 Suppl):S117-20.

[52] Dunser MW, Hasibeder WR, Wenzel V, Schwarz S, Ulmer H, Knotzer H, et al. Endocrinologic response to vasopressin infusion in advanced vasodilatory shock. *Crit Care Med.* 2004 Jun;32(6):1266-71.

[53] Choong K, Kissoon N. Vasopressin in Pediatric Shock and Cardiac arrest. *Pediatr Crit Care Med.* 2008;9:372-9.

[54] Kam P, Williams S, Yoong F. Vasopressin and terlipressin: pharmacology and its clinical relevance. *Anaesthesia.* 2004;59:993-1001.

[55] Morelli A, Ertmer C, Rehberg S, Lange M, Orecchioni A, Cecchini V, et al. Continuous terlipressin versus vasopressin infusion in septic shock (TERLIVAP): a randomized, controlled pilot study. *Crit Care.* 2009;13(4):R130.

[56] Papoff P, Mancuso M, Barbara C, Moretti C. Papoff P, Mancuso M, Barbara CS, Moretti C. *Int J Immunopathol Pharmacol.* 2007;20(2):213-21.

[57] Zeballos G, López-Herce J, Fernández C, Brandstrup K, Rodríguez-Núñez A. Rescue therapy with terlipressin by continuous infusion in a child with catecholamine-resistant septic shock. *Resuscitation.* 2006;68(1):151-3.

[70] Martin S, Yule D, Dunne M, Gallacher D, Petersen O. Vasopressin directly closes ATP-sensitive potassium channels evoking membrane depolarization and an increase in the free intracellular Ca concentration in insulin-secreting cells. *EMBO J.* 1989;8:3595-9.

[71] d'Emmanuele di Villa Bianca R, Lippolis L, Autore G, Popolo A, Marzocco S, Sorrentino R. Dexamethasone improves vascular hyporeactivity induced by LPS in vivo by modulating ATP-sensitive potassium channels activity. *Br J Pharmacol* 2003;140:91-6.

[72] Murasawa S, Matsubara H, Kizima K, Maruyama K, Mori Y, Inada M. Glucocorticoids regulate V1a vasopressin receptor expression by increasing mRNA stability in vascular smooth muscle cells. *Hypertension.* 1995;26:665-9.

[73] Russell JA, Walley KR, Gordon A, Cooper D, Hebert P, Singer J, et al. Interaction of vasopressin infusion, corticosteroid treatment and mortality of septic shock. *Crit Care Med.* 2009;37:811-8.

[74] Torgersen C, Dunser MW, Wenzel V, Jochberger S, Mayer V, Schmittinger C, et al. Comparing two different arginine vasopressin doses in advanced vasodilatory shock: a randomized controlled, open-label trial. *Intensive Care Med.* 2009;36:57-65.

[75] Lauzier F, Lesur O. Arginine-vasioressin and corticosteroids in septic shock: engaged but not yet married! *Intensive Care Med.* 2011;37:1406-8.

[76] Morris D, Dereczyk B, Grzybowski M, Martin G, Rivers E, Wortsman J, et al. Vasopressin can increase coronary perfusion pressure during human cardiopulmonary resuscitation. *Acad Emerg Med.* 1997;4(9):878-83.

[77] Lindner K, Dirks B, Strohmenger H, Prengel A, Lindner I, Lurie K. Randomised comparison of epinephrine and vasopressin in patients with out-of-hospital ventricular fibrillation. *Lancet.* 1997;349(9051):535-7.

[78] Stiell I, Hébert P, Wells G, Vandemheen K, Tang A, Higginson L, et al. Vasopressin versus epinephrine for inhospital cardiac arrest: a randomised controlled trial. *Lancet.* 2001;358(9276):105-9.

[79] Wenzel V, Kirsmer A, Arntz H, Sitter H, Stadlbauer K, Lindner K. A comparison of vasopressin and epinephrine for out-of-hospital cardiopulmonary resuscitation. *NEJM.* 2004;350(2):105-13.

[80] Aung K, Htay T. Vasopressin for Cardiac Arrest. *Arch Intern Me* 2005;165:17-24.

[58] Rehberg S, Ertmer C, Lange M, Morelli A, Whorton E, Dunser M, Role of selective V2-receptor-antagonism in septic shock: a random controlled, experimental study. *Crit Care*. 2010;14:R200.

[59] Maybauer M, Maybauer D, Enkhbaatar P, Traber D. Physiolog vasopressin receptors. *Best Pract Res Clin Anaesthesiol.* 2008;22 63.

[60] Doepker B, Lucarelli M, Lehman A, Shirk M. Thromboembolic e during continuous vasopressin infusions; a retrospective evaluation *Pharmacother*. 2007;41:1383-9.

[61] Lange M, Morelli A, Ertmer C, Koehler G, Broking K, Hucklenbru Continuous versus bolus infusion of terlipressin in ovine endotox *Shock*. 2007;28:623-9.

[62] Albanese L, Leone M, Delmas A, Martin C. Terlipressi norepinephrine in hyperdynamic septic shock: a prospective randon study. *Crit Care Med.* 2005;33:1897-902.

[63] Lauzier F, Levy B, Lamarre P, Lesur O. Vasopressin or norepinep in early hyperdynamic septic shock: a randomized controlled cli trial. *Intensive Care Med.* 2006;32:1782-9.

[64] Malay MB, Ashton RC, Jr., Landry DW, Townsend RN. Low vasopressin in the treatment of vasodilatory septic shock. *J Tra* 1999 Oct;47(4):699-703; discussion -5.

[65] Morelli A, Ertmer C, Lange M, Dunser M, Rehberg S, Van Aken al. Effects of short-term simulataneous infusion of dobutamine terlipressin in patients with septic shock: the DOBUPRESS study. *Anaesth* 2008;100:494-503.

[66] Russell J, Walley K, Singer J, Gordon A, Hebert P, Cooper J, Vasopressin versus norepinephrine infusion in patients with s shock. *NEJM*. 2008;358(9):877-87.

[67] Russell J, Walley K, Singer J, Gordon A, Hebert P, Copper J, Vasopressin versus norepinephrine infusion in patients with s shock. *New Engl J Med.* 2008;358(9):877-87.

[68] Polito A, Parisini E, Ricci Z, Picardo S, Annane D. Vasopressin fo treatment of vasodilatory shock: an ESICM systematic review and r analysis. *Intensive Care Med*. 2012;38:9-19.

[69] Weidenfeld J, Yirmiya R. Effects of bacterial endotoxin on glucocorticoid feedback regulation of adrenocortical response to st *Neuroimmunomodulation*. 1996;3:352-7.

[81] Meyer S, McGuire W, Gottschling S, Shamdeen G, Gortner L. The role of vasopressin and terlipressin in catecholamine-resistant shock and cardio-circulatory arrest in children: Review of the literature. *Wien Med Wochenschr.* 2011;161(7-8):192-203.

[82] Meyer S, Gortner L, McGuire W, Baghai A, Gottschling S. Vasopressin in catecholamine-refractory shock in children *Anaesthesia.* 2008;63:228-34.

[83] Meyer S. Vasopressin infusion therapy for refractory hypotension in extremely low birthweight neonates. Pediatrics international : *official journal of the Japan Pediatric Society.* [Comment Letter]. 2011 Apr;53(2):287.

[84] Yildizdas D, Yapicioglu H, Celik U, Serdemir Y, Alhan E. Terlipressin as a rescue therapy for catecholamine-resistant septic shock in children. *Intensive Care Med.* 2008;34:511-7.

[85] Voelckel W, Lurie K, McKnite S, Zielinski T, Lindstrom P, Peterson C, et al. Comparison of epinephrine and vasopressin in a pediatric porcine model of asphyxial cardiac arrest. *Crit Care Med.* 2000;28(12):3777-83.

[86] Voelckel W, Lurie K, McKnite S, Zielinski T, Lindstrom P, Peterson C, et al. Effects of epinephrine and vasopressin in a piglet model of prolonged ventricular fibrillation and cardiopulmonary resuscitation. *Crit Care Med.* 2002;30(5):957-62.

[87] Duncan J, Schexnayder S, Goel R, Simpson P, Bird T, Robbins J, et al. Vasopressin for in-hospital pediatric cardiac arrest: results from the AHA National Registry for CPR (NRCPR). *Pediatr Crit Care Med.* 2009;10(12):191-5.

[88] Ertmer C, Rehberg S, Westphal M. Vasopressin analogues in the treatment of shock states: potential pitfalls. *Best Practice & Research Clinical Anaesthesiology.* 2008;22(2):393-406.

[89] Choong K, Joffe A, Menon K, Fraser D, McNamara P, Litalien C, et al. Vasopressin in Pediatric Vasodilatory Shock Trial. *Am J Respir Crit Care Med.* 2009;180:632-9.

[90] Dellinger R, Levy M, Carlet J, Parker M, Jaeschke R, Reinhart K, et al. Surviving Sepsis Campaign: International guidelines for management of severe sepsis and septic shock. *Crit Care Med.* 2008;36(1):296-327.

[91] Vasu T, Cavallazzi R, Hirani A, Kaplan G, Leiby B, Marik P. Norepinephrine or dopamine for septic shock: systematic review of randomized clinical trial. *J Intensive Care Med.* 2012;27(3):172-8.

[92] Aneja R, Carcillo J. Differences between adult and pediatric septic shock. *Minerva Anestesiol.* 2011;77(10):986-92.

[93] Brierley J, Carcillo J, Choong K, Cornell T, Decaen A, Deymann A, et al. Clinical practice parameters for hemodynamic support of pediatric and neonatal septic shock: 2007 update from the American College of Critical Care Medicine. *Crit Care Med.* 2009;37:666-88.

[94] Yildizdas D, Ozden Ozgur H, Erdem S. Beneficial effects of Terlipressin in Pediatric Cardiac Arrest. *Pediatric Emergency Care.* 2011;27(9):865-8.

[95] Alten J, Borasino S, Toms R, Law M, Moellinger A, Dabal R. Early initiation of arginine vasopressin infusion in neonates after complex cardiac surgery. *Pediatr Crit Care Med.* 2012;13(3):300-4.

[96] Agrawal A, Singh V, Varma A, Sharma R. Intravenouse Arginine Vasopressin Infusion in Refractory Vasodilatory Shock: A Clinical Study. *Indian J Pediatr.* 2012;79(4):488-93.

[97] Meyer S, Löffler G, Polcher T, Gottschling S, Gortner L. Vasopressin in catecholamine-resistant septic and cardiogenic shock in very-low-birthweight infants. *Acta Paediatr.* 2006;95(10):1309-12.

[98] Rodriguez-Nunez A, Lopez-Herce J, Gil-Anton J, Hernandez A, Rey C. Rescue treatment with terlipressin in children with refractory septic shock: a clinical study. *Crit Care.* [Multicenter Study Research Support, Non-U.S. Gov't]. 2006 Feb;10(1):R20.

[99] Gil-Antón J, López-Herce J, Morteruel E, Carrillo A, Rodríguez-Núñez A. Pediatric cardiac arrest refractory to advanced life support: is there a role for terlipressin? *Pediatr Crit Care Med.* 2010;11(1):139-41.

[100] Mann K, Berg R, Nadkarni V. Beneficial effects of vasopressin in prolonged pediatric cardiac arrest: a case series. *Resuscitation.* 2002;52:149-56.

In: Vasopressin
Editor: Leonzio Galella
ISBN: 978-1-62417-311-0

Chapter 3

THE THERAPEUTIC POTENTIAL AND THE CHALLENGES OF MODULATING MYOMETRIAL SMOOTH MUSCLE TONE THROUGH THE VASOPRESSIN V_{1A} RECEPTOR

Nick Pullen[*]
Pfizer Global Research and Development,
Cambridge, MA, US

ABSTRACT

Arginine vasopressin plays a key role in the regulation of diverse physiological processes in the cardiovascular, renal, uterine and CNS systems. Abnormal release or activation of vasopressin receptors appears to contribute to the disease pathogenesis and physiology of a number of conditions including polycystic kidney disease, congestive heart failure, septic shock and depression, especially.

In recent years, both improved biophysical techniques as well as the discovery of potent and selective vasopressin ligands have helped facilitate a better understanding of the critical receptors involved in these disease processes. Here I will outline the role of vasopressin in the regulation of normal myometrial smooth muscle contraction during menstruation and parturition as well as the consequences of inappropriate activation leading to dysmenorrhoea and early labour.

[*] Email: dr.nick.pullen@gmail.com.

INTRODUCTION

Arginine vasopressin (AVP) is a cyclical nonapeptide which is principally synthesized in the neurosecretory cells of the paraventricular and supraoptic nuclei of the hypothalamus and stored in the posterior pituitary gland. Oxytocin is often co-expressed and co-released at sites of AVP synthesis. For both hormones, their plasma secretion is stimulated by oestrogen and inhibited by progestagens.

There is also evidence that AVP and oxytocin are synthesized in the periphery as well, for instance during foetal development, the foetus can also produce substantial amounts of vasopressin and oxytocin. Additionally, the uterus itself may be an important source of these hormones.

In the CNS, AVP functions as a neurotransmitter on centrally expressed vasopressin V_{1A} and V_{1B} receptors, mediating adrenocorticopin release on pituitary cortiocotrophs as well as additional behavioural and endocrine responses triggered by anxiety and stress [1].

The pathophysiological consequences of deregulated AVP secretion have been studied in a large number of systems especially renal and cardiac. For the context of this review, I will concentrate on what is known about the role of AVP in regulating uterine and vascular smooth muscle systems. In recent years, a class of vasopressin receptor antagonists, the 'vaptans' has emerged as an important class of agents [2, 3] with potential benefit in treating dysmenorrhoea, pre-term labour, hyponatremia, congestive heart failure and polycystic kidney disease. Within this class, most clinical progress has been made with the group of vasopressin V_2 receptor antagonists, exemplified by tolvaptan and conivaptan, for congestive heart failure and polycystic kidney disease agents [2, 3, 4].

The development of selective agents has been challenging due to both the peptidic nature of the ligand, the high receptor homology between vasopressin V_{1A}, V_{1B} and V_2 receptors as well as others (e.g. oxytocin receptor) and the challenges of engineering orthologous pharmacological activity for broad clinical efficacy and safety testing.

For agents which can modulate the vasopressin V_{1A} receptor specifically, there has been some notable success in recent years [5, 6, 7] and I will discuss how the in vitro and in vivo characterization of these compounds has led to greater understanding of the role of AVP in regulating normal and pathophysiological processes in gyneacology.

ROLE OF VASOPRESSIN IN REGULATION OF MYOMETRIAL TONE

Several gynaecological conditions appear to be as a consequence of altered or inappropriate myometrial contractility; these include pre-term labour and primary dysmenorrhoea. Pre-term labour is defined as the onset of labour prior to 37 weeks of gestation and is the single most important cause of perinatal mortality and morbidity in high-income countries. The pathophysiology is not well understood and often multifactorial; initiating factors include intrauterine infection, inflammation, ischemia, over-distension, and hemorrhage. While infection plays a substantial role in the genesis of pre-term labour, tocolytics such as the once approved β-adrenoceptor-2 agonist drugs, terbutaline and riordrine, fenoterol, the Ca^{2+}-channel blocker, nifedipine, and the oxytocin and vasopressin V_{1A} receptor antagonist, atosiban, have been developed and used to delay labour to a critical period to improve neonatal outcome and allow corticosteroids to be given to help the baby's lungs and other organs to mature.

The pituitary and foetal release of oxytocin and vasopressin is under the influence of ovarian steroids. The two hormones stimulate uterine contractions in pregnant and non-pregnant women via myometrial oxytocin and vasopressin V_{1A} receptors. While there may be an increase in the pulse frequency at the onset of labour, maternal plasma concentrations of oxytocin and/or vasopressin do not appear to rise significantly. Both in vitro as well as in vivo studies in pre-clinical models and humans have emphasized the importance of both ligands in the regulation of myometrial tone [8-12]. However, as both oxytocin and vasopressin appear to contribute to myometrial smooth muscle contraction and both ligands have affinity for either receptor, dissecting the specific role for either receptor has been challenging. [11, 13, 14].

In contrast, primary dysmenorrhoea is a common gynaecological complaint. Primary dysmenorrhea is defined as recurrent, crampy pain occurring with menses in the absence of identifiable pelvic pathology. The mechanisms of primary dysmenorrhoea are unclear, but both the terminal luteal phase decrease in progesterone levels and elevation in uterine prostaglandin concentrations, on the first day of bleeding, have been strongly implicated. Symptoms are manifested at a time of markedly increased myometrial activity and ischemia caused by associated reduction in uterine blood flow [15, 16]. This myometrial activity is modulated and augmented by prostaglandin synthesis. Uterine contractions can last many minutes and may produce uterine pressures of greater than 60 mmHg. The use of glyceryl trinitrate or treatment with agents which relax myometrial smooth muscle have underscored the importance of uterine tone and vascular blood flow changes in women with primary dysmenorrhoea [17, 18]. Hypercontractility and dysperistalsis of the uterus are believed to increase intrauterine pressure, leading to diminished blood flow in uterine vessels and tissue ischemia contributing to pain [18, 19]. In support of this hypothesis, Doppler and MRI studies have shown alterations in myometrial vascularization and vessel resistance during the early menstrual phases in women with dysmenorrhoea compared with women without pain [20-23]. These observations of uterine hypercontractility and dysperistalsis also appear to hold true for woman with pre-term labour and recurrent miscarriage.

It is from the seminal work of the late Scandinavian gynecologist, Mats Åkerlund, and later replicated by others, that vasopressin was first identified as a potentially important regulator of myometrial contractility under these circumstances [8, 19, 24-28]. Vasopressin levels appear to be raised in women with dysmenorrhoea both prior to and during menstruation [16, 19, 29, 30], the effects of which appear to increase myometrial smooth muscle contraction [25, 30]. The role of AVP in regulating myometrial activity has been especially emphasized from experimental studies conducted in women with moderate to severe primary dysmenorrhoea. These studies have been conducted in a number of different ways. Firstly either direct injection or haemostatic elevation of vasopressin by a bolus of hypotonic saline has been shown to increase intrauterine pressure (Figure 1) in healthy volunteers [19, 31] and facilitate pain in women with primary dysmenorrhoea (Figure 2). It has been noted, and this may be important in the context of the latter commentary in this chapter, that the effects of vasopressin on myometrial contraction and increased interuterine pressure are not synchronous with the appearance of dysmenorrhoeic pain.

Combined oral contraceptive (COC) or NSAIDs, such as naproxen, are commonly prescribed for the treatment of moderate to severe primary dysmenorrhoea. Before the availability of selective vasopressin receptor antagonists, several early studies indicated that the beneficial effects of COCs and NSAIDs were in part mediated by altering the myometrial response to vasopressin. For instance, Ekstrom et al [19, 27] demonstrated that COCs reduced the response on intrauterine pressure and contractility alone to an exogenously administered AVP and $PGF_{2\alpha}$ challenge compared with the previous baseline (Figure 3).

Expression and in vitro pharmacology studies have indicated that oxytocin and vasopressin V_{1A} receptors are functionally expressed on human myometrial [5, 9, 10, 13, 34-36], blood vessel [37, 38] and endometrial tissue [39].

Several classes of agents have been discovered, developed and tested in recent years to test the hypothesis that blockade of oxytocin and/or vasopressin V_{1A} receptors could inhibit uterine myometrial contraction and have utility in the treatment of dysmenorrhoea. The first among these that was studied was the peptide analogue atosiban (1-deamino-2-D-Tyr(OEt)-4-Thr-8-Orn-oxytocin) a moderately selective vasopressin V_{1A} receptor and oxytocin receptor antagonist. Atosiban is highly effective at reducing myometrial tone in vitro and reducing uterine contractility in vivo [10, 40-42], and given these properties it was specifically developed as a tocolytic. Its clinical benefit, however, has been considerably less than had been anticipated. Recent Cochrane analyses [43, 44] have failed to demonstrate the superiority of atosiban over betamimetics or placebo in terms of tocolytic efficacy or infant outcomes given as an intravenous agent immediately or as a maintenance regimen. Similar disappointing outcome findings in threatened pre-term labour have also been observed with barusiban, a selective oxytocin receptor antagonist with greater potency and longer duration of action than atosiban [45]. There remains a considerably high unmet medical need for preventive therapies for pre-term labour. Only the calcium channel blocker, nifedipine, appears to have a better neonatal outcome and fewer maternal side-effects than beta-mimetics, and nifedipine is also known to be teratogenic, limiting its clinical utility.

In studies performed by the Åkerlund group [25, 30], intravenously administered atosiban has been shown to decrease visual-analogue (VAS) scale pain scores and intrauterine pressure induced by vasopressin in patients with primary dysmenorrhoea or healthy subjects. These data and clinical development of atosiban, as a tocolytic approach for pre-term labour, fuelled the quest for novel orally active and selective agents for gynecological conditions. The human vasopressin V_{1A} receptor has presented a considerable challenge to the identification of potent and selective antagonists, however a marked turning point was the discovery of OPC-21268, 1-[1-[4-(3-acetlyaminopropoxy(benzoyl]-4-piperidyl)-3,4-dihydro-2(i*H*)-quinolinone [46]. While OPC-2168 lacked affinity for the human vasopressin V_{1A} receptor, its discovery enabled the identification of SR-49059 (relcovaptan; (2S) 1-[2R, 3S]-5-chloro-3-(2-chlorophenyl)-1-(3,4-dimethoxybenzeme-sulphonyl)-3-hydroxy-2,3-dihydro-1H-indole-2-carbonyl]-pyrolidinone-2-carboxamide; [7]), an orally bioavailable and potent vasopressin V_{1A} receptor antagonist with greater than 100 fold selectivity over vasopressin V_{1B}, V_2 and oxytocin receptors.. In the study of the regulation of myometrial contraction, SR-49059 has been an important tool. Using a similar paradigm as that used to evaluate atosiban, the Åkerlund group were able to show that SR-49059 was able to reduce vasopressin-induced myometrial contractions [8, 9]. These data have been used to build confidence in additional small clinical studies, to determine the effect of SR-49059 on myometrial contractions in women with pre-term labour and primary dysmenorrhoea. In women with pre-term labour (weeks 32–36), an oral dose of SR-49059 (400 mg) reduced uterine contractions from 8.2±1.4 to 3.2±0.9 contractions/30 mins compared with 9.7±1.6 to 7.8±2.2/30 mins measured by external tocodynamometry [47]. Studies evaluating SR-49059 on pregnancy outcome have not been conducted.

In the only other double-blind, randomised, placebo-controlled, cross-over clinical study of its type, conducted by the Åkerlund group [26], SR-49059 (100 and 300 mg) was assessed for effect on menstrual pain, as recorded by visual analogue scale, in women with primary dysmenorrhoea. Compared with placebo, SR-49059 (300 mg) reduced the VAS pain score by approximately 20%, a magnitude of effect which would be comparable with NSAIDs. For an agent that supposedly would directly attenuate myometrial and uterine artery contraction, the magnitude of effect might be considered a little disappointing compared with the therapeutic objective. However, the possibility that the 300 mg dose did not achieve sufficient receptor occupancy can be inferred by interpolating the exposure data and from studies conducted with higher doses. Interpolation of exposures suggests that 300 mg dose achieved exposures which were a relatively modest multiple of the Ki value for the human vasopressin V_{1A} receptor. Supporting this notion are observations from the studies described above when a 400 mg dose was tested in women with pre-term labour [47]. In this study, there was a larger magnitude of effect of SR-49059 on uterine contractions than that observed from vasopressin-infusion studies [8, 9].

While SR-49059 is no longer in clinical development, several other agents have been identified including VA-111913 [48], PF-00738245 [5], YM-218 [49], SRX-246/251 and JNJ-17308616 [6]. Building on the initial observations made with SR-49059, anyone of these agents might be anticipated to have a beneficial effect in primary dysmenorrhoea. Of these, VA-111913 is currently the farthest in development having reportedly completed PhIIa clinical assessment in patients with primary dysmenorrhoea (ClinicalTrials.gov identifier: NCT00963053). According to company disclosures, VA-111913 was well tolerated in the study and statistically significant differences between

VA-111913 treatment and placebo were seen for a number of efficacy endpoints, including treatment preference, and a trend to efficacy was seen in all other relevant endpoints. However, that the study did not meet its primary endpoints suggests that either study design, dose or inclusion criteria were not optimal or that only a sub-population of individuals had benefit from VA-111913 treatment.

Despite the observation of elevated vasopressin associated with dysmenorrhoea and the recognition that vasopressin, through the vasopressin V_{1A} receptor, appears to regulate myometrial tone, we are clearly a long way from a deep understanding of the pathophysiology of primary dysmenorrhoea and further research is needed to understand this.

So far the anticipated benefits of selectively targeting the vasopressin V_{1A} receptor have not yielded sufficient promise as a treatment for primary dysmenorrhoea.

Rodent studies have indicated that the vasopressin V_{1A} receptor also appears to play a role in the regulation of numerous social and behavioral processes such as aggression, social bonding and anxiety. The potential benefits of targeting the CNS expressed vasopressin V_{1A} receptor in primary dysmenorrhoea, however, have been somewhat overlooked eventhough the condition is associated with high levels of anxiety.

As there are no pre-clinical models of dysmenorrhoeic pain, information on the potential role for vasopressin has been evaluated in a number of anxiety models.

In rats and hamsters, blocking the vasopressin V_{1A} receptor by destruction of AVP-expressing olfactory neurons or pharmacological blockade alters maternal aggression and reduces anxiety-like behaviour [6, 50-54].

There have been considerable challenges in development of CNS penetrant vasopressin V_{1A} receptor antagonists and a recent analysis of the available chemical substrate, including VA-111913, suggests that few disclosed examples are anticipated to have considerable CNS penetration [55].

This then may be an additional unexplored factor in the clinical assessment of vasopressin V_{1A} receptor antagonists for primary dysmenorrhoea; the absence of anticipated CNS exposure of VA-111913, atosiban and SR-49059 reducing the potential anxiolytic benefit in the patient population.

POTENTIAL CLINICAL UTILITY OF VASOPRESSIN V_{1A} RECEPTOR ANTAGONISTS IN OTHER GYNEACOLOGICAL CONDITIONS

The potential therapeutic utility of vasopressin receptor V_{1A} antagonists has so far not been realized in the treatment of pre-term labour and primary dysmenorrhoea and despite the clinical precedence that has been set by agents such as atosiban.

There are two other areas of emerging clinical interest which are worthy of note in the context of the effects of vasopressin in the treatment of gyneacological conditions. These are as a supplement to assisted reproduction therapy (ART) and endometriosis.

Despite tremendous progress in assisted reproduction technology over the past few decades, the overall effectiveness of even the most advanced treatments is still relatively low, averaging about 30% live births per treatment cycle. While a lot of attention has been focused on embryo quality, the process of embryo transfer and the environment is being increasingly recognized as being important [56, 57].

A large proportion of embryos are lost during the transfer process. Uterine hypercontractility and dysperistalsis may constitute one of the most fundamental components of uterine receptivity and embryo retention. As the expression of oxytocin and vasopressin V_{1A} receptors responds to changes in ovarian hormone levels, it might be anticipated that this expression would persist in response to supraphysiological concentrations of oestradiol which accompany an ART cycle. This might be expected to alter uterine contractility and indeed, it has been shown that uterine contractile activity increases approximately six-fold during an ART cycle compared with the baseline cycle [58].

The evidence that a vasopressin V_{1A} receptor antagonist has potential utility as part of the ART/IVF cycle has come from several clinical studies using atosiban [59]. In the first reported outcome, atosiban was successfully administered to a 42-year-old woman who had previously undergone 8 embryo transfers, a 15 year history of infertility. For this case, the infusion of atosiban caused a decrease in the frequency and magnitude of uterine contractions during embryo transfer and resulted in successful normal twin diamniotic pregnancy [59]. More recently, a Turkish group [60] has reported on a randomized, placebo controlled study evaluating the effects of an intravenous dose of atosiban on pregnancy and implantation rate following embryo transfer to 160 women. In this report the pregnancy and implantation rates per embryo transfer were 46.7% and 20.4% in the atosiban-treated group, compared with 28.9% and 12.6%, respectively, in the control group. Furthermore, the miscarriage rate observed in the atosiban treated group was 16.7% compared with 24.4%, in the control group. There are no reported studies with any oral non-peptide vasopressin receptor antagonists, such as SR-49059. While the potential teratogenic implications of these sorts of assessments on the developing embryo need to be very cautiously examined, so far the data generated with atosiban are encouraging and warrant further investigation.

Finally I would like to highlight some considerations for the potential utility of vasopressin receptor V_{1A} antagonists in the treatment of endometriosis. Endometriosis is a benign condition characterised by the ectopic growth of endometrial glandular and stromal tissue outside the uterine cavity, especially on the ovaries, the Pouch of Douglas and peritoneum. The conditions presents with infertility, dysmenorrhoeic as well as chronic pelvic pain and menorrhagia. It is not clear what the origins of dysmenorrhoeric pain are or, indeed, whether the vasopressin axis plays a similar role in secondary dysmenorrhoea as has been anticipated from studies of primary dysmenorrhoea.

One of the founding theories on the disease pathogenesis is the Sampson hypothesis of retrograde menstruation [61]. In support of the theory are the observations of altered uterine peristalsis in woman with endometriosis [62-64], potentially limiting directed sperm transport and high fundal implantation, contributing to infertility, as well as serving retrograde menstruation for the preservation of body iron content.

Furthermore, it has become apparent that the ectopic lesions also express vasopressin V_{1A} and oxytocin receptors [39, 65] and their expression may also directly contribute to the disease condition and persistence.

In support of the latter observations, recently a Turkish group [66] have described the effects of atosiban (0.5 mg/kg/day) given intraperitoneally on the growth of ectopic endometriotic lesions in a rat model of endometriosis. They found that atosiban reduced the volume of ectopic implants by approximately 30% compared with a vehicle control group.

Whilst the data require independent replication, the notion that a vasopressin/oxytocin receptor antagonist as well as potentially reducing retrograde menstruation and reducing dysmenorrhoeic pain, might also directly influence the growth of endometriotic lesions is intriguing.

Safety Implications of Vasopressin V_{1A} Receptor Antagonism

Vasopressin V_{1A} receptors are widely expressed on the vasculature, and, as described above, one of the anticipated effects of vasopressin on the vessels which supply the myometrium is to cause vessel constriction, ischemia and dysmenorrhoea. Indeed, the vascular expression of vasopressin V_{1A} receptors has prompted the development of vasopressin V_{1A} receptor agonists, such as FE 202158, for the prevention of vasodilatory hypotension associated with septic shock [67]. One of the earliest observations of the use of OPC-22158 and SR-49059 in healthy volunteers [8, 47, 68, 69] was the ability of vasopressin V_{1A} receptor antagonists to inhibit the vasoconstrictor response to infused AVP or CGRP. This has been widely reproduced in multiple systems and has been used to build confidence in the pharmacology of these agents for the purposes of dose setting and confirming receptor engagement [5]. As vasopressin V_{1A} receptors are expressed in the renal macula densa, this suggests a role in renin-angiotensin production. Based on these observations, one of the projected downsides of chronic exposure of selective vasopressin V_{1A} receptor antagonists could be the potential to cause hypotension, a hypothesis which is consistent with the observed effects in knockout animals [70-73]. Consistent with this, a decrease in blood pressure has been noted in some chronic dosing studies with SR-49059 [8, 24, 47], but not others [26]. Vasopressin V_{1A} receptors are also expressed on platelets, where they contribute to platelet aggregation in response to AVP. In vitro and ex vivo studies with SR-49059 for instance, have shown that SR-49059 can block AVP-induced platelet aggregation [7, 74]. Further studies are required to better understand the cardiovascular consequences, for instance the potential for orthostatic hypotension and clotting effects in the target patient population treated with vasopressin V_{1A} receptor antagonists.

Conclusion

While the discovery of OPC-22158 was a cornerstone in the identification and development of the selective, orally bioavailable vasopressin V_{1A} receptor antagonist SR-49059, the clinical studies performed by Åkerlund group put the potential importance of the vasopressin V_{1A} receptor in regulation myometrial tone on the map. It is fair to say, however, that, despite this considerable achievement, the full therapeutic potential of vasopressin V_{1A} receptor antagonists in the treatment of gynecological conditions such as dysmenorrhoea, endometriosis and pre-mature labour has not been fully acceded. This may be in part due to the regulatory environment and caution that needs to be headed when conducting clinical studies and treatment of women of child-bearing potential. Additionally the Pharma appetite and activity in Women's Health has been declining in recent years as a result of great organizational transformation and consolidation in the sector.

The effects of vasopressin on eliciting myometrial smooth muscle contraction have been clearly demonstrated from in vitro and in vivo studies [5, 7, 8, 24]. An unambiguous role for the vasopressin V_{1A} receptor in mediating the contraction of uterine vascular and tissue smooth muscle contraction has been concluded from these studies. However, if therapeutic utility is dependent on describing with certainty the relationship to a pathological condition, then certainly there is also a strong case for oxytocin in mediating a similar effect on uterine myometrium. In both cases, the causal relationship between altered vasopressin and oxytocin signaling and disease pathogenesis has not been rigorously confirmed. For instance, metaanalyses conducted on the clinical benefit of atosiban in the prevention of pre-term labour, have not fully supported the notion that suppressing myometrial contraction results in a significant clinical benefit. A similar case has been presented for the treatment of primary dysmenorrhoea; uterine and, presumably, uterine artery contraction are reduced in the presence of a vasopressin V_{1A} receptor antagonists, but the anticipated improvement in symptoms has neither been unambiguously demonstrated nor appears to be superior to that acceded by COX inhibition. For dysmenorrhoea, this may be, in part, due to compensation by oxytocinergic pathways or the requirement to target CNS expressed vasopressin V_{1A} receptors. Whilst further research is needed to better understand disease causality in pre-term labour and primary dysmenorrhoea, there are considerable challenges in clinical evaluation in these disease areas and the translational value of pre-clinical models is not clear either. Despite these risks and uncertainly, here appears to be continuing interest in the modulation of the vasopressin V_{1A} receptor. For instance in endometriosis or as a supplement to ART, as described above, but additionally, the expression of vasopressin V_{1A} receptors on vascular smooth muscle has highlighted the involvement on AVP in propagating the abnormal vasoactive response in Raynaud's syndrome [75]. The development of SR-49059 was curtailed for undisclosed reasons, but was apparently safe and well tolerated in the clinical assessments which had been conducted. While the discovery of CNS penetrant vasopressin V_{1A} receptor antagonists still presents a considerable medicinal chemistry challenge [55], the identification of agents such as VA-111913 and PF-00738245 [5] represents a potentially important step forward in realizing therapeutic value in this area.

REFERENCES

[1] Egashira N, Mishima K, Iwasaki K, Oishi R, Fujiwara M (2009) New topics in vasopressin receptors and approach to novel drugs: role of the vasopressin receptor in psychological and cognitive functions. *J. Pharmacol. Sci.* 109: 44-49.

[2] Favory R, Salgado DR, Vincent J-L (2009) Investigational vasopressin receptor modulators in the pipeline. *Expert Opinion on Investigational Drugs* 18: 1119-1131.

[3] Veeraveedu PT, Palaniyandi SS, Yamaguchi Ki, Komai Y, Thandavarayan RA, et al. (2010) Arginine vasopressin receptor antagonists (vaptans): pharmacological tools and potential therapeutic agents. *Drug Discovery Today* 15: 826-841.

[4] Ambrosy A, Goldsmith SR, Gheorghiade M (2011) Tolvaptan for the treatment of heart failure: a review of the literature. *Expert Opin. Pharmacother* 12: 961-976.

[5] Russell R, Doyle R, Turner J, Attkins N, Ramsey S, et al. (2011) In vitro and in vivo pharmacological characterisation of the potent and selective vasopressin V(1A) receptor antagonist 4-[4-(4-Chloro-phenyl)-5-[1,2,3]triazol-2-ylmethyl-4H-[1,2,4]triazol-3-yl]-piperi din-1-yl-(3,5-difluoro-phenyl) methanone (PF-00738245). *Eur. J. Pharmacol.* 670: 347-355.

[6] Bleickardt CJ, Mullins DE, Macsweeney CP, Werner BJ, Pond AJ, et al. (2009) Characterization of the V1a antagonist, JNJ-17308616, in rodent models of anxiety-like behavior. *Psychopharmacology* (Berl) 202: 711-718.

[7] Serradeil-Le Gal C, Wagnon J, Garcia C, Lacour C, Guiraudou P, et al. (1993) Biochemical and pharmacological properties of SR 49059, a new, potent, nonpeptide antagonist of rat and human vasopressin V1a receptors. *J. Clin. Invest* 92: 224-231.

[8] Bossmar T, Brouard R, Doberl A, Akerlund M (1997) Effects of SR 49059, an orally active V1a vasopressin receptor antagonist, on vasopressin-induced uterine contractions. *Br. J. Obstet. Gynaecol.* 104: 471-477.

[9] Bossmar T, Rasmussen T, Akerlund M (1996) Effect of the non-peptide, vasopressin V1a receptor antagonist, SR 49059 and its enantiomer, SR 49770, on isolated human myometrium. *Acta Obstet Gynecol. Scand* 75: 516-519.

[10] Wilson RJ, Allen MJ, Nandi M, Giles H, Thornton S (2001) Spontaneous contractions of myometrium from humans, non-human primate and rodents are sensitive to selective oxytocin receptor antagonism in vitro. *BJOG* 108: 960-966.

[11] Bossmar T, Akerlund M, Fantoni G, Szamatowicz J, Melin P, et al. (1994) Receptors for and myometrial responses to oxytocin and vasopressin in preterm and term human pregnancy: effects of the oxytocin antagonist atosiban. *Am. J. Obstet. Gynecol* 171: 1634-1642.

[12] Akerlund M (2002) Involvement of oxytocin and vasopressin in the pathophysiology of preterm labor and primary dysmenorrhea. *Prog. Brain Res.* 139: 359-365.

[13] Bossmar T, Akerlund M, Szamatowicz J, Laudanski T, Fantoni G, et al. (1995) Receptor-mediated uterine effects of vasopressin and oxytocin in nonpregnant women. *Br. J. Obstet Gynaecol.* 102: 907-912.

[14] Akerlund M, Bossmar T, Brouard R, Kostrzewska A, Laudanski T, et al. (1999) Receptor binding of oxytocin and vasopressin antagonists and inhibitory effects on isolated myometrium from preterm and term pregnant women. *Br. J. Obstet Gynaecol.* 106: 1047-1053.

[15] Akerlund M (1994) Vascularization of human endometrium. Uterine blood flow in healthy condition and in primary dysmenorrhoea. *Ann. N. Y Acad Sci.* 734: 47-56.

[16] Stromberg P, Akerlund M, Forsling ML, Granstrom E, Kindahl H (1984) Vasopressin and prostaglandins in premenstrual pain and primary dysmenorrhea. *Acta Obstet. Gynecol. Scand* 63: 533-538.

[17] Pittrof R, Lees C, Thompson C, Pickles A, Martin JF, et al. (1996) Crossover study of glyceryl trinitrate patches for controlling pain in women with severe dysmenorrhoea. *BMJ* 312: 884.

[18] Akerlund M, Andersson KE, Ingemarsson I (1976) Effects of terbutaline on myometrial activity, uterine blood flow, and lower abdominal pain in women with primary dysmenorrhoea. *Br. J. Obstet Gynaecol.* 83: 673-678.

[19] Ekstrom P, Akerlund M, Forsling M, Kindahl H, Laudanski T, et al. (1992) Stimulation of vasopressin release in women with primary dysmenorrhoea and after oral contraceptive treatment--effect on uterine contractility. *Br. J. Obstet. Gynaecol.* 99: 680-684.

[20] Altunyurt S, Gol M, Sezer O, Demir N (2005) Primary dysmenorrhea and uterine blood flow: a color Doppler study. *J. Reprod. Med.* 50: 251-255.

[21] Dmitrovic R, Peter B, Cvitkovic-Kuzmic A, Strelec M, Kereshi T (2003) Severity of symptoms in primary dysmenorrhea--a Doppler study. *Eur. J. Obstet Gynecol. Reprod. Biol.* 107: 191-194.

[22] Royo P, Alcazar JL (2008) Three-dimensional power Doppler assessment of uterine vascularization in women with primary dysmenorrhea. *J. Ultrasound. Med.* 27: 1003-1010.

[23] Kataoka M, Togashi K, Kido A, Nakai A, Fujiwara T, et al. (2005) Dysmenorrhea: evaluation with cine-mode-display MR imaging--initial experience. *Radiology* 235: 124-131.

[24] Steinwall M, Bossmar T, Gaud C, Akerlund M (2004) Inhibitory effects of SR 49059 on oxytocin-and vasopressin-induced uterine contractions in non-pregnant women. *Acta Obstet Gynecol Scand* 83: 12-18.

[25] Liedman R, Grant L, Igidbashian S, James I, McLeod A, et al. (2006) Intrauterine pressure, ischemia markers, and experienced pain during administration of a vasopressin V1a receptor antagonist in spontaneous and vasopressin-induced dysmenorrhea. *Acta Obstet Gynecol Scand* 85: 207-211.

[26] Brouard R, Bossmar T, Fournie-Lloret D, Chassard D, Akerlund M (2000) Effect of SR49059, an orally active V1a vasopressin receptor antagonist, in the prevention of dysmenorrhoea. *BJOG* 107: 614-619.

[27] Ekstrom P, Juchnicka E, Laudanski T, Akerlund M (1989) Effect of an oral contraceptive in primary dysmenorrhea--changes in uterine activity and reactivity to agonists. *Contraception* 40: 39-47.

[28] Valentin L, Sladkevicius P, Kindahl H, Broeders A, Marsal K, et al. (2000) Effects of a vasopressin antagonist in women with dysmenorrhea. *Gynecol Obstet Invest* 50: 170-177.

[29] Hauksson A, Akerlund M, Forsling ML, Kindahl H (1987) Plasma concentrations of vasopressin and a prostaglandin F2 alpha metabolite in women with primary dysmenorrhoea before and during treatment with a combined oral contraceptive. *J. Endocrinol.* 115: 355-361.

[30] Hauksson A, Akerlund M, Melin P (1988) Uterine blood flow and myometrial activity at menstruation, and the action of vasopressin and a synthetic antagonist. *Br. J. Obstet Gynaecol.* 95: 898-904.

[31] Liedman R, Skillern L, James I, McLeod A, Grant L, et al. (2006) Validation of a test model of induced dysmenorrhea. *Acta Obstet Gynecol. Scand* 85: 451-457.

[32] Tahara A, Saito M, Sugimoto T, Tomura Y, Wada K, et al. (1998) Pharmacological characterization of the human vasopressin receptor subtypes stably expressed in Chinese hamster ovary cells. *Br. J. Pharmacol.* 125: 1463-1470.

[33] Schoneberg T, Kostenis E, Liu J, Gudermann T, Wess J (1998) Molecular aspects of vasopressin receptor function. *Adv. Exp. Med. Biol.* 449: 347-358.

[34] Liedman R, Hansson SR, Howe D, Igidbashian S, Russell RJ, et al. (2008) Endometrial expression of vasopressin, oxytocin and their receptors in patients with primary dysmenorrhoea and healthy volunteers at ovulation. *Eur. J. Obstet Gynecol Reprod Biol.* 137: 189-192.

[35] Thornton S, Baldwin PJ, Harris PA, Harding F, Davison JM, et al. (2002) The role of arginine vasopressin in human labour: functional studies, fetal production and localisation of V1a receptor mRNA. *BJOG* 109: 57-62.

[36] Pettibone DJ, Clineschmidt BV, Lis EV, Reiss DR, Totaro JA, et al. (1991) In vitro pharmacological profile of a novel structural class of oxytocin antagonists. *J. Pharmacol. Exp. Ther.* 256: 304-308.

[37] Kostrzewska A, Laudanski T, Steinwall M, Bossmar T, Serradeil-Le Gal C, et al. (1998) Effects of the vasopressin V1a receptor antagonist, SR 49059, on the response of human uterine arteries to vasopressin and other vasoactive substances. *Acta Obstet Gynecol Scand* 77: 3-7.

[38] Jovanovic A, Grbovic L, Zikic I, Tulic I (1995) Characterization of arginine vasopressin actions in human uterine artery: lack of role of the vascular endothelium. *Br. J. Pharmacol* 115: 1295-1301.

[39] Mechsner S, Grum B, Gericke C, Loddenkemper C, Dudenhausen JW, et al. (2010) Possible roles of oxytocin receptor and vasopressin-1alpha receptor in the pathomechanism of dysperistalsis and dysmenorrhea in patients with adenomyosis uteri. *Fertil Steril* 94: 2541-2546.

[40] Bossmar T (1998) Treatment of preterm labor with the oxytocin and vasopressin antagonist Atosiban. *J. Perinat. Med.* 26: 458-465.

[41] Nilsson L, Reinheimer T, Steinwall M, Akerlund M (2003) FE 200 440: a selective oxytocin antagonist on the term-pregnant human uterus. *BJOG* 110: 1025-1028.

[42] Goodwin TM, Paul R, Silver H, Spellacy W, Parsons M, et al. (1994) The effect of the oxytocin antagonist atosiban on preterm uterine activity in the human. *Am. J. Obstet. Gynecol.* 170: 474-478.

[43] Papatsonis D, Flenady V, Cole S, Liley H (2005) Oxytocin receptor antagonists for inhibiting preterm labour. *Cochrane Database Syst. Rev*: CD004452.

[44] Papatsonis D, Flenady V, Liley H (2009) Maintenance therapy with oxytocin antagonists for inhibiting preterm birth after threatened preterm labour. *Cochrane Database Syst Rev*: CD005938.

[45] Thornton S, Goodwin TM, Greisen G, Hedegaard M, Arce JC (2009) The effect of barusiban, a selective oxytocin antagonist, in threatened preterm labor at late gestational age: a randomized, double-blind, placebo-controlled trial. *Am. J. Obstet. Gynecol.* 200: 627 e621-610.

[46] Yamamura Y, Ogawa H, Chihara T, Kondo K, Onogawa T, et al. (1991) OPC-21268, an orally effective, nonpeptide vasopressin V1 receptor antagonist. *Science* 252: 572-574.

[47] Steinwall M, Bossmar T, Brouard R, Laudanski T, Olofsson P, et al. (2005) The effect of relcovaptan (SR 49059), an orally active vasopressin V1a receptor antagonist, on uterine contractions in preterm labor. *Gynecol Endocrinol* 20: 104-109.

[48] Batt AR, Heeney CMS (2011) 1,4-Disubstituted piperidines as vasopressin receptor V1A antagonists. US 2011/0312941 A1.

[49] Tsukada J, Tahara A, Tomura Y, Kusayama T, Wada K, et al. (2005) Pharmacologic properties of YM218, a novel, potent, nonpeptide vasopressin V1A receptor-selective antagonist. *Vascul Pharmacol* 42: 47-55.

[50] Tobin VA, Hashimoto H, Wacker DW, Takayanagi Y, Langnaese K, et al. (2010) An intrinsic vasopressin system in the olfactory bulb is involved in social recognition. *Nature* 464: 413-417.

[51] Ferris CF, Lu SF, Messenger T, Guillon CD, Heindel N, et al. (2006) Orally active vasopressin V1a receptor antagonist, SRX251, selectively blocks aggressive behavior. *Pharmacol. Biochem. Behav.* 83: 169-174.

[52] Caffrey MK, Nephew BC, Febo M (2010) Central vasopressin V1a receptors modulate neural processing in mothers facing intruder threat to pups. *Neuropharmacology* 58: 107-116.

[53] Bosch OJ, Neumann ID (2008) Brain vasopressin is an important regulator of maternal behavior independent of dams' trait anxiety. *Proc. Natl. Acad. Sci. USA* 105: 17139-17144.

[54] Bosch OJ, Neumann ID (2010) Vasopressin released within the central amygdala promotes maternal aggression. *Eur. J. Neurosci.* 31: 883-891.

[55] Ryckmans T (2010) Modulation of the vasopressin system for the treatment of CNS diseases. *Curr. Opin. Drug Discov. Devel.* 13: 538-547.

[56] Tomas C, Tikkinen K, Tuomivaara L, Tapanainen JS, Martikainen H (2002) The degree of difficulty of embryo transfer is an independent factor for predicting pregnancy. *Hum. Reprod.* 17: 2632-2635.

[57] Fanchin R, Ayoubi JM (2009) Uterine dynamics: impact on the human reproduction process. *Reprod Biomed Online* 18 Suppl 2: 57-62.

[58] Ayoubi JM, Epiney M, Brioschi PA, Fanchin R, Chardonnens D, et al. (2003) Comparison of changes in uterine contraction frequency after ovulation in the menstrual cycle and in in vitro fertilization cycles. *Fertil Steril* 79: 1101-1105.

[59] Pierzynski P, Reinheimer TM, Kuczynski W (2007) Oxytocin antagonists may improve infertility treatment. *Fertil Steril* 88: 213 e219-222.

[60] Moraloglu O, Tonguc E, Var T, Zeyrek T, Batioglu S (2010) Treatment with oxytocin antagonists before embryo transfer may increase implantation rates after IVF. *Reprod. Biomed Online* 21: 338-343.

[61] Sampson JA (1927) Metastatic or Embolic Endometriosis, due to the Menstrual Dissemination of Endometrial Tissue into the Venous Circulation. *Am. J. Pathol* 3: 93-110 143.

[62] Kissler S, Hamscho N, Zangos S, Wiegratz I, Schlichter S, et al. (2006) Uterotubal transport disorder in adenomyosis and endometriosis--a cause for infertility. *BJOG* 113: 902-908.

[63] Leyendecker G, Kunz G, Wildt L, Beil D, Deininger H (1996) Uterine hyperperistalsis and dysperistalsis as dysfunctions of the mechanism of rapid sperm transport in patients with endometriosis and infertility. *Hum. Reprod.* 11: 1542-1551.

[64] Salamanca A, Beltran E (1995) Subendometrial contractility in menstrual phase visualized by transvaginal sonography in patients with endometriosis. *Fertil Steril* 64: 193-195.

[65] Barcena de Arellano ML, Gericke J, Reichelt U, Okuducu AF, Ebert AD, et al. (2011) Immunohistochemical characterization of endometriosis-associated smooth muscle cells in human peritoneal endometriotic lesions. *Hum. Reprod.* 26: 2721-2730.

[66] Simsek Y, Celik O, Karaer A, Gul M, Yilmaz E, et al. (2012) Therapeutic efficiency of Atosiban, an oxytocin receptor blocking agent in the treatment of experimental endometriosis. *Arch. Gynecol. Obstet* 10.1007/s00404-012-2390-7 [doi].

[67] Laporte R, Kohan A, Heitzmann J, Wisniewska H, Toy J, et al. (2011) Pharmacological characterization of FE 202158, a novel, potent, selective, and short-acting peptidic vasopressin V1a receptor full agonist for the treatment of vasodilatory hypotension. *J. Pharmacol. Exp. Ther* 337: 786-796.

[68] Imaizumi T, Harada S, Hirooka Y, Masaki H, Momohara M, et al. (1992) Effects of OPC-21268, an orally effective vasopressin V1 receptor antagonist in humans. *Hypertension* 20: 54-58.

[69] Weber R, Pechere-Bertschi A, Hayoz D, Gerc V, Brouard R, et al. (1997) Effects of SR 49059, a new orally active and specific vasopressin V1 receptor antagonist, on vasopressin-induced vasoconstriction in humans. *Hypertension* 30: 1121-1127.

[70] Fujisawa Y, Miyatake A, Hayashida Y, Aki Y, Kimura S, et al. (1994) Role of vasopressin on cardiovascular changes during hemorrhage in conscious rats. *Am. J. Physiol* 267: H1713-1718.

[71] Aoyagi T, Izumi Y, Hiroyama M, Matsuzaki T, Yasuoka Y, et al. (2008) Vasopressin regulates the renin-angiotensin-aldosterone system via V1a receptors in macula densa cells. *Am. J. Physiol. Renal Physiol* 295: F100-107.

[72] Aoyagi T, Koshimizu TA, Tanoue A (2009) Vasopressin regulation of blood pressure and volume: findings from V1a receptor-deficient mice. *Kidney Int.* 76: 1035-1039.

[73] Koshimizu TA, Nasa Y, Tanoue A, Oikawa R, Kawahara Y, et al. (2006) V1a vasopressin receptors maintain normal blood pressure by regulating circulating blood volume and baroreflex sensitivity. *Proc. Natl. Acad. Sci. USA* 103: 7807-7812.

[74] Brouard R, Laporte V, Serradeil Le Gal C, Pignol R, Jang H, et al. (1998) Safety, tolerability, and pharmacokinetics of SR 49059, a V1a vasopressin receptor antagonist, after repeated oral administration in healthy volunteers. *Adv. Exp. Med. Biol.* 449: 455-465.

[75] Hayoz D, Bizzini G, Noel B, Depairon M, Burnier M, et al. (2000) Effect of SR 49059, a V1a vasopressin receptor antagonist, in Raynaud's phenomenon. *Rheumatology* (Oxford) 39: 1132-1138.

In: Vasopressin
Editor: Leonzio Galella

ISBN: 978-1-62417-311-0

Chapter 4

THE EFFICACY OF VASOACTIVE MEDICATIONS IN ACUTE VARICEAL BLEEDS

Malcolm Wells*[*]*, Nilesh Chande and Melanie Beaton
Schulich School of Medicine and Dentistry,
Western University,
London, ON, Canada

ABSTRACT

Vasoactive medications such as vasopressin, somatostatin and their analogues are commonly used for the treatment of acute variceal bleeding. Vasoactive medications have been used for over thirty years and management has improved with better endoscopic therapies and the use of antibiotics prophylactically.

Even with such a long history, the risks and benefits of the use of vasoactive medications continue to be debated. In this article we explore the evidence behind the efficacy of these medications.

* Corresponding author: Malcolm Wells MD, 339 Windermere Road, PO Box 5339, London, Ontario, Canada N6A 5A5, Telephone: (519) 685-8500, Email: mwells22@uwo.ca.

INTRODUCTION

Acute esophageal variceal bleeding is an important cause of morbidity and mortality in patients with cirrhosis [1-6]. Current treatment strategies, that include vasoactive medications, have resulted in improved survival [1, 3, 7]. Treatment options include administration of vasoactive pharmacological agents, endoscopic variceal banding or sclerotherapy, balloon tamponade, transjugular intrahepatic portosystemic stenting and surgery. Two classes of vasoactive pharmacological agents for have been evaluated for the treatment of acute variceal bleeding [8, 9]: vasopressin and its analogues, and somatostatin and its analogues. Vasopressin is the most potent splanchnic vasoconstrictor, reducing blood flow to splanchnic organs, thereby leading to a decrease in portal venous inflow and a decrease in portal pressures. There is concern regarding side effects of cardiac, peripheral and bowel ischemia related to its potent vasoconstrictive properties [10].

Although concomitant administration of nitrates improves efficacy and reduces adverse ischemic events [11], these complications still are more prevalent with vasopressin than other vasoactive agents [12] limiting the utility of this agent. Vasopressin is administered at a continuous IV infusion of 0.2-0.4 units/minute that can be increased to a maximal dose of 0.8 units/minute. It can only be used continuously at maximal dose for 24 hours in order to minimize the development of side effects. It should always be accompanied by IV nitroglycerin at a starting dose of 40μg/minute, which can be increased to a maximum of 400μg/minute, adjusted to maintain a systolic blood pressure 90mmHg [8, 9]. Terlipressin (triglycyl lysine vasopressin) is an analogue of vasopressin that has longer biological activity and fewer cardiac, bowel and peripheral ischemic side effects [8, 9].

It can be administered by intermittent intravenous injections rather than by continuous infusion. Whereas a small study demonstrated a rapid increase in the plasma level of the fibrinolytic proenzyme plasminogen activator in patients receiving vasopressin, no such fibrinolytic response was found with terlipressin [13], which theoretically means terlipressin doesn't disrupt clot formation as vasopressin may. Terlipressin is administered at an initial dose of 2 mg IV every 4 hours and can be titrated down to 1 mg IV every 4 hours once hemorrhage is controlled [14].

Somatostatin, and its analogues octreotide and vapreotide, cause splanchnic vasoconstriction due to inhibition of the release of vasodilatory peptides, mainly glucagon. Octreotide also has a local vasoconstrictive effect

[12, 15, 16]. These agents are relatively safe in comparison to vasopressin and can be used continuously for 5 days or longer allowing treatment during the period at which the risk of rebleeding is highest. Octreotide is the most commonly used vasoactive medication. It is typically used as an initial IV bolus of 50 mcg followed by a continuous infusion of 50 μg/hour. Use of somatostatin consists of a 250μcg IV bolus followed by infusion of 250μcg/hour. Vapreotide is given as a 50μcg IV bolus followed by infusion of 50 μcg per hour [8, 9].

American Association of the Study of Liver Diseases (AASLD) guidelines recommend pharmacological therapy (somatostatin or its analogues octreotide and vapreotide; terlipressin) should be initiated as soon as variceal hemorrhage is suspected and continued for 3-5 days after diagnosis is confirmed (Class I, Level A) [8, 9]. This review will discuss the evidence demonstrating the efficacy of somatostatin, vasopressin and their analogues in the treatment of acute variceal bleeds.

Comparison of Vasoactive Medications with Control

Mortality

Several early randomized controlled trials and meta-analyses investigating the efficacy of vasoactive pharmacological agents versus placebo control in patients with acute esophageal bleeds, were not able to identify a mortality benefit [17-27].

Ioannou and colleagues performed a Cochrane Review in 2003 (updated in 2009) that first identified a mortality benefit with terlipressin in acute variceal bleeds [28, 29]. In seven randomized, placebo-controlled trials with a total of 443 patients compared to placebo, terlipressin led to a significant reduction in mortality (relative risk of 0.66, 95% confidence interval (CI) 0.49–0.88).

Follow-up in the seven trials ranged from 5 to 42 days. Variceal bleeding is immediately life threatening, however these patients have underlying disease that carries a large mortality risk in the longer term. Thus, the efficacy of treatment with vasoactive agents for an acute life-threatening variceal bleed is more accurately gauged by differences in 5- to 7-day mortality, whereas 42-day mortality rates may reflect the severity of the underlying cirrhosis.

Wells *et al* (2012) performed a meta-analysis where they investigated the early 7-day mortality and intermediate 30-day mortality in acute esophageal variceal bleeding treated with vasoactive medications versus placebo [30]. It is the first and only meta-analysis to demonstrate vasoactive medications significantly reduce the risk of all-cause seven-day mortality as compared with placebo (19 studies; risk ratio (RR) 0.74, 95% confidence interval (CI) 0.57-0.95; P=0.02; I^2=0%).

The risk of intermediate all-cause mortality at 8-42 days trended towards a beneficial effect in patients treated with vasoactive agents compared with the control group (n=20; RR 0.80, 0.64-1.00; P=0.05; I^2=21%). The conclusions of this systematic review are limited by the poor to moderate quality of supporting evidence, and the publication dates ranging from 1978 to 2008. Over that 30-year period routine standard of care improved and mortality decreased.

Hemostasis

Multiple meta-analyses have found there to be a significant increase in hemostasis with the use of vasoactive medications. In a meta-analyses by Gøtzsche [26, 27], the number of patients failing initial haemostasis was reduced in a meta-analyses by relative risk 0.68 (0.54 to 0.87). Compared to placebo, terlipressin led to significant reductions in failure of initial haemostasis (relative risk of 0.66, 95% CI 0.53–0.82; 7 RCT's; total patients 443) [31]. When combined, vasoactive agents were associated with a significant increase in hemostasis (n=25; RR 1.21, 95% CI 1.13-1.30; P<0.001; I^2=27%) [30].

Rebleeding

Multiple Randomized Controlled Trials (RCT's) and meta-analyses demonstrate a decrease in rebleeding with vasoactive medications. Among them are Corley's meta-analysis, that demonstrated significantly less rebleeding from octreotide vs. placebo/no intervention (all patients received sclerotherapy/band ligation before randomization to placebo vs. octreotide) (RR, 0.46; 95% CI, 0.32-0.67; test for homogeneity, P = 0.4) [25]. A meta-analysis by Wells *et al* found the risk of rebleeding was statistically significantly lower (16 trials; risk ratio of 0.68; 0.52 to 0.90; P=0.007;

I^2=41%) in patients treated with vasoactive agents versus control [30]. Multiple other meta-analyses demonstrate similar results [26-29, 32]. In contrast, in a meta-analyses by Gøtzsche [26, 27], the number of patients with rebleeding was not significantly reduced for the trials with a low risk of bias, relative risk 0.84 (0.52 to 1.37) while it was substantially reduced in the other trials, relative risk 0.36 (0.19 to 0.68).

Transfusion Requirements

RCT's and meta-analyses consistently demonstrate vasoactive agents significantly decrease transfusion requirements. Meta-analyses by Gøtzsche [26, 27], Ioannou [28, 29, 31], Wells [30] all demonstrated significantly fewer units of packed red blood cells were required. In general, most meta-analyses found a decrease in 0.7 units were required when vasoactive medications were given as compared to placebo. Although statistically significant, it is questionable if 0.7 units has clinically significance.

Hospital Stay

The length of hospital stay was significantly lower in patients treated with vasoactive agents than with control when Wells et al (2012) pooled patients from three studies, with a mean difference of -0.71 (-1.23 to -0.19; P=0.007; I^2=0%) [30].

Limitations

There are limitations to all the meta-analyses performed. Many of the randomized trials were small, low quality, unblinded studies. In addition, some of the outcomes commonly used, such as control of bleeding and rebleeding, are relatively subjective and therefore may be subject to ascertainment bias, especially in non-blinded studies [33]. Despite the development of consensus statements [34], most studies have used divergent definitions of control of bleeding and rebleeding, which makes it even harder to make direct comparisons. Finally, some argue that it may be misleading to group vasopressin, somatostatin and their analogues together as those vasoactive medications have slightly different mechanisms of action [6, 13].

Table 1. Dosing of Vasoactive Medications

Medication	Initial Dose	Maximum Dose
Vasopressin +/- nitroglycerin	0.2 units/minute IV infusion +/- Nitroglycerin 40 mg/min	0.8 units/minute IV infusion +/- Nitroglycerin 400 mg/min
Terlipressin	1-2mg IV q4 hours	1-2mg IV q4 hours
Somatostatin	250mcg IV bolus followed by 250mg/h IV infusion	250mcg IV bolus followed by 250mg/h IV infusion
Octreotide	25-50 mcg IV bolus followed by 25-50mcg/h IV infusion	50 mcg IV bolus followed by 50mcg/h IV infusion
Vapreotide	50 mcg/h IV infusion	50 mcg/h IV infusion

Comparison of Effect between Vasoactive Medications

There have been a handful of trials and meta-analyses comparing the various vasoactive medications head-to-head.

Corley et al (2001) performed a meta-analysis comparing octreotide to other pharmaceutical therapies. There was no evidence of a survival benefit from octreotide compared with vasopressin/terlipressin (RR, 0.80; 95% CI, 0.54-1.19; test for homogeneity, P = 0.88). Patients receiving octreotide versus vasopressin/terlipressin had significantly reduced rebleeding (RR, 0.58; 95% CI, 0.42-0.81; test for homogeneity, P = 0.97). Octreotide had fewer major complications than vasopressin/terlipessin (RR, 0.31; 95% CI, 0.11-0.87), and a complication profile comparable to no intervention/placebo (RR, 1.06; 95% CI, 0.72-1.55). No specific alternative therapy demonstrated a mortality benefit.

The second meta-analysis compared octreotide, terlipressin, somatostatin, and vasopressin to each other [30]. Comparisons of terlipressin with somatostatin, terlipressin with vasopressin, octreotide with terlipressin, and octreotide with somatostatin failed to demonstrate a significant difference in mortality, hemostasis and rebleeding. There was significantly greater hemostasis with use of octreotide when compared to vasopressin (n=2; RR 1.31, CI 1.10-1.56) whereas mortality was not significantly different (n=1; RR 1.00, CI 0.54-1.85). Hemostasis was significantly lower with vasopressin when compared with somatostatin (n=6; RR 0.75, CI 0.61-0.92) whereas no significant difference in mortality or rebleeding was detectable.

Comparison of Effect between Vasoactive Medications and Endoscopic Therapy

In a meta-analysis by Corley and colleagues (2001), Octreotide had comparable efficacy to immediate sclerotherapy for control of bleeding (RR, 0.94; 95% CI, 0.55-1.62) [25]. Overall mortality at the end of follow-up was not decreased significantly by octreotide compared with alternative pharmacologic or mechanical interventions (i.e., sclerotherapy, band ligation, or balloon tamponade) (RR, 0.89; 95% confidence interval [CI], 0.7-1.14; test for homogeneity, P = 0.3).

Ioannou *et al* (2003) performed a meta-analyses that, in part, compared terlipressin and endoscopic sclerotherapy (EST) [31]. They found no significant differences in mortality, failure of hemostasis, rebleeding and additional procedures for uncontrolled bleeding, when comparing terlipressin with EST (1 high quality trial analyzed).

D'Amico et al has published three Cochrane Reviews on the comparison of EST versus vasoactive medications in variceal bleeding [14, 35, 36]. In the latest review [36], seventeen trials including 1817 patients were identified. No significant differences were found in any outcome when comparing EST with vasopressin (1 trial), terlipressin (1 trial), somatostatin (5 trials), and octreotide (10 trials). Combining all the trials irrespective of the vasoactive drug, the risk differences (95% confidence intervals) were failure to control bleeding -0.02 (-0.06 to 0.02), five-day failure rate -0.05 (-0.10 to 0.01), rebleeding 0.01 (-0.03 to 0.05), mortality (17 randomised trials, 1817 patients) -0.02 (-0.06 to 0.02), and transfused blood units (8 randomised trials, 849 patients) (weighted mean difference) -0.24 (-0.54 to 0.07). Adverse events 0.08 (0.03 to 0.14) and serious adverse events 0.05 (0.02 to 0.08) were significantly more frequent with EST.

There are limitations to the comparisons of sclerotherapy to vasoactive medications for acute variceal bleeding, as EST is no longer the preferred endoscopic therapy. The American Society for Gastrointestinal Endoscopy (ASGE) recommends the use of endoscopic variceal ligation (EVL), rather than EST, as the endoscopic treatment of choice for controlling esophageal variceal hemorrhage and for secondary variceal obliteration [37]. This was based on six randomized prospective trials [38-43] and one meta-analysis [44], that showed superiority of EVL over EST for all major outcomes including recurrent bleeding, local complications including ulceration and stricture formation, time to variceal obliteration, and survival. Complications of EST include fever, retrosternal discomfort or pain, dysphagia, injection-induced bleeding, esophageal ulceration with delayed bleeding, esophageal perforation, mediastinitis, pleural effusion, bronchoesophageal fistula, adult respiratory distress syndrome, and infectious complications [45, 46]. In contrast to EST, EVL appears to rarely induce bacteremia but has poor efficacy on gastric varices.

In addition, common practice dictates and guidelines recommend the combination of both pharmacological and endoscopic therapy for acute esophageal variceal bleeding. The AASLD Practice Guideline recommends vasoactive medications to be initiated as soon as variceal hemorrhage is suspected and continued for 3-5 days after diagnosis is confirmed, as well as endoscopic treatment to be performed within 12 hours (Class I, Level A) [8, 9]. A meta-analysis of 8 trials involving 939 patients demonstrated that combined treatment improved initial control of bleeding (relative risk [RR], 1.12; 95% confidence interval (CI), 1.02-1.23; NNT 8), and 5-day hemostasis (RR, 1.28; 95% CI, 1.18-1.39; NNT 5). Mortality was not significantly decreased by combined therapy (RR, 0.73; 95% CI, 0.45-1.18). Severe adverse events were similar in both groups [47].

Comparison of Effect between Vasoactive Medications and Balloon Tamponade

The meta-analysis by Ioannou *et al* (2003) compared terlipressin and balloon tamponade [31]. Analysis of 3 low-quality studies comparing terlipressin with balloon tamponade yielded no significant difference in overall mortality, failure of hemostasis, and rebleeding.

For multiple reasons, direct comparison of vasoactive medications and balloon tamponade has little clinical significance. First, balloon tamponade is usually implemented as a rescue after failure of vasoactive medications and endoscopic treatment, or in severe cases of hemorrhage. In these patients both vasoactive medications and balloon tamponade therapy would be occurring concomitantly.

Secondly, while balloon tamponade is very effective in controlling bleeding immediately in over 80% of patients [48], it does have its limitations and is not a first line therapy. Balloon tamponade is associated with potentially lethal complications such as aspiration, migration, and necrosis/perforation of the esophagus with mortality rates as high as 20% [8, 9]. AASLD guidelines recommend balloon tamponade should be restricted to use as a temporizing measure for a maximum of 24 hours in patients with uncontrollable bleeding for whom a more definitive therapy (e.g., TIPS or endoscopic therapy) is planned (Class I, Level B) [8, 9].

Discussion and Conclusion

Summary of Evidence

With over 50 RCT's and multiple meta-analyses over more than 30 years, there is significant evidence supporting the now common use of vasoactive medications in acute variceal bleeding. The use of vasoactive agents was associated with a significantly lower risk of acute 7-day mortality and, in the case of terlipressin, decreased 5-42 day mortality. There is also a great deal of evidence for significant improvement in hemostasis, rebleeding, lower transfusion requirements, and a shorter hospital stay. Studies comparing different vasoactive agents have not shown a clinically significant difference in effect. Studies and meta-analyses show comparable results with vasoactive medications and endoscopic therapy or balloon tamponade, however it is now common practice to use these interventions together.

Implications for Clinical Practice

Vasoactive agents have become the standard of care in the treatment of acute variceal bleeding. Present evidence exists for a reduction in acute mortality rate, rebleeding, transfusion requirements, and hospital stay and an improvement in hemostasis. At the current time, there is sufficient evidence to recommend the use of vasoactive agents in clinical practice and as reflected in current guidelines [8, 9].

Implications for Research

The current practice of administering vasoactive medications in patients undergoing acute variceal bleeds is supported by the current evidence, but it is not clear whether one agent is superior to another. Furthermore, there is little evidence regarding the use of a combination of vasoactive agents. A methodologically rigorous randomized controlled trial of the combination of two vasoactive agents, powered to detect a difference in clinically relevant outcomes would further clarify the benefits and risks of the current standards of care in the management of patients with acute variceal bleeding.

ACKNOWLEDGMENTS

The authors would like to thank Dr. Paul Adams for his help in editing the manuscript.

Competing Interest Statement

All authors have completed the Unified Competing Interest form at http://www.icmje.org/coi_disclosure.pdf (available on request from the corresponding author).

REFERENCES

[1] Carbonell N, Pauwels A, Serfaty L, Fourdan O, Levy VG, Poupon R. Improved survival after variceal bleeding in patients with cirrhosis over the past two decades. *Hepatology*. 2004 Sep;40(3):652-9.

[2] Chalasani N, Kahi C, Francois F, Pinto A, Marathe A, Bini AJ. Improved patient survival after acute variceal bleeding: a multicenter, cohort study. *American Journal of Gastroenterology*. 2003;98:653-9.

[3] D'Amico G, De Franchis R. Upper digestive bleeding in cirrhosis. Post-therapeutic outcome and prognostic indicators. *Hepatology*. [Multicenter Study; Research Support, Non-U.S. Gov't]. 2003 Sep;38(3):599-612.

[4] Graham DY, Smith JL. The course of patients after variceal hemorrhage. *Gastroenterology*. 1981 Apr;80(4):800-9.

[5] Sorbi D, Gostout CJ, Peura D, Johnson D, Lanza F, Foutch PG, et al. An assessment of the management of acute bleeding varices: a multicenter prospective member-based study. Am J Gastroenterol. [Comparative Multicenter Study]. 2003 Nov;98(11):2424-34.

[6] Burroughs AK. Pharmacological treatment of acute variceal bleeding. *Digestion*. [Review]. 1998 Jul;59 Suppl 2:28-36.

[7] Chalasani N, Kahi C, Francois F, Pinto A, Marathe A, Bini EJ, et al. Improved patient survival after acute variceal bleeding: a multicenter, cohort study. *Am J Gastroenterol.* [Multicenter Study; Research Support, Non-U.S. Gov't; Research Support, U.S. Gov't, P.H.S.]. 2003 Mar;98(3):653-9.

[8] Garcia-Tsao G, Sanyal AJ, Grace ND, Carey WD. Prevention and management of gastroesophageal varices and variceal hemorrhage in cirrhosis. *Am J Gastroenterol.* [Practice Guideline]. 2007 Sep;102(9):2086-102.

[9] Garcia-Tsao G, Sanyal AJ, Grace ND, Carey W. Prevention and management of gastroesophageal varices and variceal hemorrhage in cirrhosis. *Hepatology*. [Practice Guideline]. 2007 Sep;46(3):922-38.

[10] Bolognesi M BG, Garcia-Tsao G, Gatta A, Gines P, Merli M, et al. , editor. Complications in the medical treatment of portal hypertension. Portal Hypertension III. . *Proceedings of the Third Baveno International Consensus Workshop on Definitions, Methodology and Therapeutic Strategies*; 2001; Oxford, UK: Blackwell Science.

[11] Groszmann RJ, Kravetz D, Bosch J, Glickman M, Bruix J, Bredfeldt J, et al. Nitroglycerin improves the hemodynamic response to vasopressin in portal hypertension. *Hepatology*. [Research Support, U.S. Gov't, P.H.S.]. 1982 Nov-Dec;2(6):757-62.

[12] D'Amico G, Pagliaro L, Bosch J. Pharmacological treatment of portal hypertension: an evidence-based approach. *Semin Liver Dis.* [Review]. 1999;19(4):475-505.

[13] Douglas JG, Forrest JA, Prowse CV, Cash JD, Finlayson ND. Effects of lysine vasopressin and glypressin on the fibrinolytic system in cirrhosis. *Gut*. 1979 Jul;20(7):565-7.

[14] D'Amico G, Pietrosi G, Tarantino I, Pagliaro L. Emergency sclerotherapy versus vasoactive drugs for variceal bleeding in cirrhosis: a Cochrane meta-analysis. *Gastroenterology*. [Comparative Study; Meta-Analysis; Research Support, Non-U.S. Gov't]. 2003 May;124(5):1277-91.

[15] Chatila R, Ferayorni L, Gupta T, Groszmann RJ. Local arterial vasoconstriction induced by octreotide in patients with cirrhosis. *Hepatology*. [Clinical Trial, Research Support, U.S. Gov't, Non-P.H.S.]. 2000 Mar;31(3):572-6.

[16] McCormick PA DR, Siringo S, et al. Octreotide reduces azygos blood flow in cirrhotic patients with portal hypertension. . *Eur J Gastroenterol Hepatol.* 1990;2:489-92.

[17] Corley D, Cello J, Adkisson W, Ko W, Kerlikowske K. Octreotide for acute esophageal variceal bleeding: a meta-analysis. *Gastroenterology*. 2001;120(4):946-54.

[18] Avgerinos A, Nevens F, Raptis S, Fevery J. Early administration of somatostatin and efficacy of sclerotherapy in acute oesophageal variceal bleeds: the European Acute Bleeding Oesophageal Variceal Episodes (ABOVE) randomised trial. *Lancet*. [Clinical Trial, Multicenter Randomized Controlled Trial, Research Support, Non-U.S. Gov't]. 1997 Nov 22;350(9090):1495-9.

[19] Besson I, Ingrand P, Person B, Boutroux D, Heresbach D, Bernard P, et al. Sclerotherapy with or without octreotide for acute variceal bleeding. *N Engl J Med.* [Clinical Trial, Multicenter Study, Randomized Controlled Trial, Research Support, Non-U.S. Gov't]. 1995 Aug 31;333(9):555-60.

[20] Burroughs AK, McCormick PA, Hughes MD, Sprengers D, D'Heygere F, McIntyre N. Randomized, double-blind, placebo-controlled trial of somatostatin for variceal bleeding. Emergency control and prevention of early variceal rebleeding. *Gastroenterology*. [Clinical Trial, Randomized Controlled Trial]. 1990 Nov;99(5):1388-95.

[21] Cales P, Masliah C, Bernard B, Garnier PP, Silvain C, Szostak-Talbodec N, et al. Early administration of vapreotide for variceal bleeding in patients with cirrhosis. *N Engl J Med.* [Clinical Trial, Multicenter Study, Randomized Controlled Trial, Research Support, Non-U.S. Gov't]. 2001 Jan 4;344(1):23-8.

[22] Fogel MR, Knauer CM, Andres LL, Mahal AS, Stein DE, Kemeny MJ, et al. Continuous intravenous vasopressin in active upper gastrointestinal bleeding. *Ann Intern Med.* [Clinical Trial, Controlled Clinical Trial, Research Support, U.S. Gov't, P.H.S.]. 1982 May;96(5):565-9.

[23] Fourtanier G, Tournut R, Clanet J, Joncquiert F, Pascal JP. [Efficacy of vasopressin in the treatment of gastrointestinal hemorrhage caused by the rupture of esophageal varices. Randomized study: preliminary results]. *Therapie.* [Clinical Trial, Randomized Controlled Trial]. 1977 May-Jun;32(3):283-6.
[24] Freeman JG, Cobden I, Record CO. Placebo-controlled trial of terlipressin (glypressin) in the management of acute variceal bleeding. *J Clin Gastroenterol.* [Clinical Trial, Controlled Clinical Trial, Randomized Controlled Trial]. 1989 Feb;11(1):58-60.
[25] Corley DA, Cello JP, Adkisson W, Ko WF, Kerlikowske K. Octreotide for acute esophageal variceal bleeding: a meta-analysis. *Gastroenterology.* [Meta-Analysis; Research Support, Non-U.S. Gov't; Research Support, U.S. Gov't, P.H.S.]. 2001 Mar;120(4):946-54.
[26] Gotzsche PC, Hrobjartsson A. Somatostatin analogues for acute bleeding oesophageal varices. *Cochrane Database Syst Rev.* [Meta-Analysis Review]. 2005(1):CD000193.
[27] Gotzsche PC, Hrobjartsson A. Somatostatin analogues for acute bleeding oesophageal varices. *Cochrane Database Syst Rev.* [Meta-Analysis; Review]. 2008(3):CD000193.
[28] Ioannou G, Doust J, Rockey DC. Terlipressin for acute esophageal variceal hemorrhage. *Cochrane Database Syst Rev.* [Review]. 2003(1):CD002147.
[29] Ioannou G, Doust J, Rockey DC. Terlipressin for acute esophageal variceal hemorrhage. *Cochrane Database Syst Rev.* [Review]. 2001(1):CD002147.
[30] Wells M, Chande N, Adams P, Beaton M, Levstik M, Boyce E, et al. Meta-analysis: vasoactive medications for the management of acute variceal bleeds. *Aliment Pharmacol Ther.* [Meta-Analysis]. 2012 Jun;35(11):1267-78.
[31] Ioannou GN, Doust J, Rockey DC. Systematic review: terlipressin in acute oesophageal variceal haemorrhage. *Aliment Pharmacol Ther.* [Research Support, Non-U.S. Gov't; Research Support, U.S. Gov't, Non-P.H.S.; Review]. 2003 Jan;17(1):53-64.
[32] Gotzsche PC. Somatostatin analogues for acute bleeding oesophageal varices. *Cochrane Database Syst Rev.* [Review]. 2002(1):CD000193.
[33] Jadad AR, Moore RA, Carroll D, Jenkinson C, Reynolds DJ, Gavaghan DJ, et al. Assessing the quality of reports of randomized clinical trials: is blinding necessary? *Control Clin Trials.* [Meta-Analysis]. 1996 Feb;17(1):1-12.

[34] de Franchis R. Updating consensus in portal hypertension: report of the Baveno III Consensus Workshop on definitions, methodology and therapeutic strategies in portal hypertension. *Journal of Hepatology.* [Research Support, Non-U.S. Gov't]. 2000 Nov;33(5):846-52.

[35] D'Amico G, Pietrosi G, Tarantino I, Pagliaro L. Emergency sclerotherapy versus medical interventions for bleeding oesophageal varices in cirrhotic patients. *Cochrane Database Syst Rev.* [Review]. 2002(1):CD002233.

[36] D'Amico G, Pagliaro L, Pietrosi G, Tarantino I. Emergency sclerotherapy versus vasoactive drugs for bleeding oesophageal varices in cirrhotic patients. *Cochrane Database Syst Rev.* [Meta-Analysis Review]. 2010(3):CD002233.

[37] Qureshi W, Adler DG, Davila R, Egan J, Hirota W, Leighton J, et al. ASGE Guideline: the role of endoscopy in the management of variceal hemorrhage, updated July 2005. *Gastrointest Endosc.* [Practice Guideline]. 2005 Nov;62(5):651-5.

[38] Stiegmann GV, Goff JS, Michaletz-Onody PA, Korula J, Lieberman D, Saeed ZA, et al. Endoscopic sclerotherapy as compared with endoscopic ligation for bleeding esophageal varices. *N Engl J Med.* [Clinical Trial Comparative Study Randomized Controlled Trial]. 1992 Jun 4;326(23):1527-32.

[39] Gimson AE, Ramage JK, Panos MZ, Hayllar K, Harrison PM, Williams R, et al. Randomised trial of variceal banding ligation versus injection sclerotherapy for bleeding oesophageal varices. *Lancet.* [Clinical Trial; Randomized Controlled Trial]. 1993 Aug 14;342(8868):391-4.

[40] Laine L, el-Newihi HM, Migikovsky B, Sloane R, Garcia F. Endoscopic ligation compared with sclerotherapy for the treatment of bleeding esophageal varices. *Ann Intern Med.* [Clinical Trial; Comparative Study; Randomized Controlled Trial]. 1993 Jul 1;119(1):1-7.

[41] Hou MC, Lin HC, Kuo BI, Chen CH, Lee FY, Lee SD. Comparison of endoscopic variceal injection sclerotherapy and ligation for the treatment of esophageal variceal hemorrhage: a prospective randomized trial. *Hepatology.* [Clinical Trial; Comparative Study; Randomized Controlled Trial; Research Support, Non-U.S. Gov't]. 1995 Jun;21(6):1517-22.

[42] Lo GH, Lai KH, Cheng JS, Hwu JH, Chang CF, Chen SM, et al. A prospective, randomized trial of sclerotherapy versus ligation in the management of bleeding esophageal varices. *Hepatology.* [Clinical Trial; Randomized Controlled Trial]. 1995 Aug;22(2):466-71.

[43] Baroncini D, Milandri GL, Borioni D, Piemontese A, Cennamo V, Billi P, et al. A prospective randomized trial of sclerotherapy versus ligation in the elective treatment of bleeding esophageal varices. *Endoscopy*. [Clinical Trial; Comparative Study; Randomized Controlled Trial]. 1997 May;29(4):235-40.

[44] Laine L, Cook D. Endoscopic ligation compared with sclerotherapy for treatment of esophageal variceal bleeding. A meta-analysis. *Ann Intern Med.* [Comparative Study; Meta-Analysis]. 1995 Aug 15;123(4):280-7.

[45] Truesdale RA, Jr., Wong RK. Complications of esophageal variceal sclerotherapy. *Gastroenterol Clin North Am.* [Review]. 1991 Dec;20(4):859-70.

[46] Edling JE, Bacon BR. Pleuropulmonary complications of endoscopic variceal sclerotherapy. *Chest.* [Review]. 1991 May;99(5):1252-7.

[47] Banares R, Albillos A, Rincon D, Alonso S, Gonzalez M, Ruiz-del-Arbol L, et al. Endoscopic treatment versus endoscopic plus pharmacologic treatment for acute variceal bleeding: a meta-analysis. *Hepatology*. [Comparative Study; Meta-Analysis; Research Support, Non-U.S. Gov't]. 2002 Mar;35(3):609-15.

[48] Avgerinos A, Armonis A. Balloon tamponade technique and efficacy in variceal haemorrhage. *Scand J Gastroenterol Suppl.* [Comparative Study; Meta-Analysis]. 1994;207:11-6.

In: Vasopressin
Editor: Leonzio Galella
ISBN: 978-1-62417-311-0

Chapter 5

Reproductive and Metabolic Responses of Desert Adapted Common Spiny Male Mice (*Acomys cahirinus*) to Vasopressin Treatment

Elena Bukovetzky, Fuad Fares, Hagit Schwimmer and Abraham Haim
Haifa University, Haifa, Israel

Abstract

Changes in day length (photoperiod) can serve as an important signal for the coming breeding season for mammals inhabiting predictable ecosystems in temperate zones. In unpredictable desert ecosystems, photoperiod changes are not a sufficient signal to predict the optimal time of breeding. Therefore, integration of various environmental cues should determine which species will be adapted to breed at the right time and to survive in xeric environments. In regards we asked the following question: What are the environmental cues and their mechanism used by xeric adapted small mammals for reproduction timing? The driving force in desert ecosystems is water and the intervals between episodes of water input into the ecosystem vary and in some years there may be no input. It has been suggested that water availability can serve as a reliable cue for reproduction.

Vasopressin (VP), a hormone involved in water balance and osmoregulation is produced by the hypothalamus and released by the neuro-pituitary. VP secretion levels increase in response to elevated plasma osmolarity, representing water shortage. VP receptors are found in the reproductive tract. The different effects of VP on metabolism and reproduction make it candidate for mediating the transmission of environmental signals to the reproductive system of desert adapted rodents. We tested the metabolic and reproductive response of males from a desert adapted population of *A. cahirinus* to VP treatment under three week acclimation to two different photoperiod regimes short (SD-8L:16D) and long (LD- 16L:8D). The results of our study show that VP treatment *per se*, caused a significant ($p<0.05$) decrease of testosterone level in SD-acclimated males. VP treatment caused an increase in FFA release of SD-acclimated males but not in LD-males. In addition, response was assessed from changes in mRNA receptor gene expression of VP (AVP) and aldosterone (nr3c2) in testis and white adipose tissue (WAT) of treated groups, compared with their control. VP treatment resulted in a decrease of VP receptor gene expression, in LD-acclimated male testis. VP caused a significant decrease in aldosteron receptor mRNA expression in SD-acclimated males, in testis, but caused its elevation in WAT. These results support the idea that water availability in the habitat may affect breeding through effects of VP, directly, on the testis, or indirectly through effects on WAT. These findings also support previous knowledge that different physiological systems could be integrated by a single hormonal signal.

INTRODUCTION

Maintenance of constant intracellular and extracellular ionic and osmotic conditions is critical for the normal functioning of cells. Osmoregulation is the process which regulates the concentration and osmotic pressure of blood by regulating the water contents of blood plasma and urine. It is an important process as excessive loss of water may cause dehydration whereas excess of water intake may dilute the body fluids [1]. One of the most important regulators in this process is vasopressin (VP). VP is an antidiuretic hormone that is produced in the cell bodies of the magnocellular neurons of the supraoptic and paraventricular nuclei in the hypothalamus. Vasopressin-releasing magnocellular neurons directly function as such osmoreceptors, responding to increased osmotic pressure in their extracellular environment by increased firing rate and concomitant vasopressin release into the circulation [2, 3]. VP is released to the blood stream from the pituitary gland, travels to the kidney and binds to membrane V2- type VP receptors in the renal collecting duct [4]. This binds resulting in the insertion of stored aquaporin (water channel) proteins into the plasma membrane and as result it triggers the contraction of the arterioles in the glomeruli and reabsorption of water from the collecting ducts. This increases water reabsorption by the kidney permitting restoration of plasma osmolality [5-7].

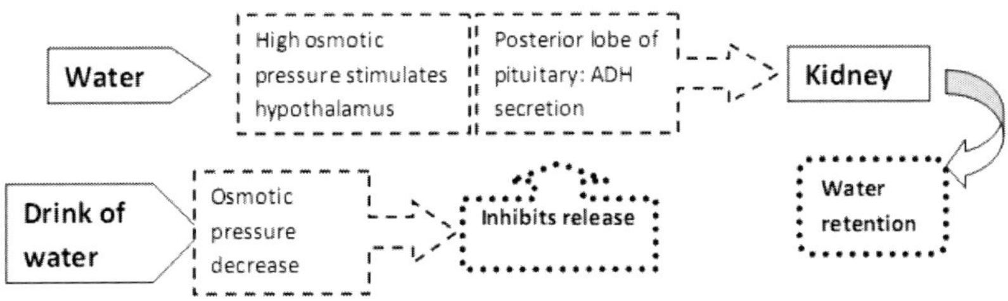

However, some recent studies learnt that VP has other peripheral effects, particularly its ability to cause a vasoconstriction of arteriolar smooth muscle, as a releasing hormone for the adenohypophysial hormone corticotrophin, and beginning to appreciate some of its central effects such as on different adaptive behaviors [8].

More recently, it has become clear that vasopressin is also synthesized in other tissues, including the sympathetic ganglia [9], the adrenals [10, 11], the ovaries [12, 13], and the testis [14, 15]. Certainly there is plenty of evidence for the presence of vasopressin receptors in all of these, and other, tissues, for example V1R in sympathetic ganglia [16], V1aR and V1bR in adrenal medulla [11, 17], V1R in heart-derived myocytes [18], V1aR, V1bR and V2R in the gastrointestinal tract [19] and V1R in the liver [20]. Schaffler et al., 2005 demonstrated the rather unexpected finding that mature adipocytes do express mRNA the specific receptors and receptor subtypes for the hypothalamic peptide vasopressin [21]. These findings certainly imply that vasopressin is a potential local autocrine regulator in many tissue systems.

VP is thought to have no direct reproductive functions [22], but recent studies hint that it may affect the reproductive system in addition to its osmoregulatory actions. In the monogamous prairie vole (*Microtus ochrogaster*) VP was found to be important for pair bonding [23, 24], and VP hypothalamic gene expression increased in both males and females postpartum [25]. The reproductive role of VP in the central nervous system is reflected in the dimorphic VP nuclei [26] and the dimorphic excretion of VP in the brain [27-29]. In rats, both VP secretion and responsiveness to VP were affected by gender and by the estrus cycle of the female [28]. In humans, plasma VP is reported lowest during and just after menstruation, when estradiol and progesterone concentrations are low and high at the time of ovulation when these hormones peak [30].

Reproduction in mammals is a highly energy consuming activity, and thus requires that the time of reproduction coincide with the time of year that the habitat is most rewarding [31]. A common cue used for triggering reproduction in predictable ecosystems with minimal year to year changes in climatic conditions is day length changes (photoperiod) [32]. However, the xeric ecosystem is defined as water-controlled, with frequent, discrete and largely unpredictable water inputs [33]. In such unpredictable ecosystems, desert species could be "misled" if they entirely rely only on photoperiod and therefore, additional cues for successful breeding are needed [34-36]. Functions such as growth and reproduction can be delayed when foraging conditions are too costly energetically, and both can be abandoned in the face of severe negative energy balance [35]. Therefore, integration of various environmental cues is an important adaptation for the optimal time of breeding and for survival in xeric environments [36].

PREVIOUS STUDIES

It was suggested earlier that osmotic stress is the major signaling pathway in desert environment and it seems likely that the reproductive system will be a strong target of natural selection when animals are in osmotically extreme environments [37, 38]. We therefore hypothesized that the reproductive system could be directly affected by factors that regulate the water balance and osmotic systems. In previous studies designed to examine the effect of increased osmotic load on physiological and endocrine parameters of desert-adapted *Acomys* population was shown a negative effect of osmotic stress on reproduction. Study was conducted on desert-adapted *A. russatus* [38, 40] and *A. cahirinus* [37, 39-40, 46] by stimulating end of summer osmotic loads by challenging the animals with a gradually increasing salinity [37-38, 40, 46] or VP injections [38-39, 45].

These damaging effects of high salinity on reproductive system (decreasing in number of estrous cycles, relative testis/ ovaries mass and sex hormone levels) were coupled with a massive (about 80%) reduction of white adipose tissue (WAT) mass in desert-adapted mice, compared with their control group [37, 40] The primary role of WAT commonly referred to as “fat” in mammals [41], is to store free fatty acids (FFA) as triglycerides (triacylglycerol) during periods of caloric excess (lipogenesis) and to mobilize these reserves and release free fatty acids for ATP synthesis via the Kreb's Cycle during periods when expenditure of calories exceeds the intake (lipolysis) [41]. WAT is now recognised as a multifunctional organ; in addition to the central role of lipid storage, it has a major endocrine function secreting several hormones, notably leptin. Clearly, the emerging picture of WAT as an endocrine and immunological organ incorporates cross-talk and co-stimulation of a multitude of hormonal signals [42]. The recent study find that matured adipocytes do express genes of specific receptors of hypothalamic VP in all three receptor subtypes V-1A, V1-B and V-2 [22, 43] Thus, WAT involvement in reproduction of desert adapted rodents is not only through secreted leptin [44] but also as a source for water supply. Our earlier results show a receptor genes expression of aldosterone (Nr3c2) and vasopressin (AVP) in both WAT and testes of *A. cahirinus* [37, 45, 46]. A strong effect of high salt treatment (ST) was noted in mRNA receptors expression genes of AVP which were significantly ($p<0.05$) increased in ST-SD females compared with their controls. Also, a significant ($p<0.05$) increase in mRNA receptor expression AVP genes was noted in under both, long and short photoperiod regimes [46].

RESULTS

These results suggest that VP could serve as a good candidate for sending the message of water shortage to the reproductive system. The accumulated knowledge so far brings us to test the following hypotheses: if VP is involved in breeding regulation of desert-adapted rodents than this hormone will have a direct effect through its receptors on the gonads or its indirect effect *via* WAT. To test these hypotheses, we examined the effects of exogenous VP, on the reproductive and metabolic activity of *A. cahirinus* males from a desert-adapted population, acclimated to SD and LD photoperiods. Treated mice were *i.p.* injected with VP solution (50 µg/kg W_b,Sigma) three times a week [39, 40], when a control group mice were *i.p.* injected with sterile saline solution (0.9%NaCl), n=6 for SD and LD- acclimated mice. Serum testosterone, leptin FFA levels were measured using ELISA, following manufacturer's instruction.

Exogenous administration of VP (50µg/Kg) for four weeks in intervals of two days did not affected W_b significantly neither in SD- nor LD-acclimated *A. cahirinus* males, but a negative effect in % of weight gain was noted: total weight gain of VP-treated males was lower, under both photoperiods, compared with their controls group (Table 1).

Table 1.

Photoperiod	Treatment	Initial W_b gr	Final W_b gr	W_b gain gr (%)
LD	Control (C)	45±2	52±2	7(15.5 %)
LD	Vasopressin (VP)	46±3	50±1.5	4 (%8)
SD	Control (C)	34±3	45±2	11 (32%)
SD	Vasopressin (VP)	35±2	42±1.4	7 (20%)

Table 2.

Treatment	LD acclimation	SD acclimation
Control (C)	0.05 nmol/μL±0.002	0.05 nmol/μL±0.003
Vasopressin (VP)	0.05 nmol/μL±0.01	0.07 nmol/μL±0.01*

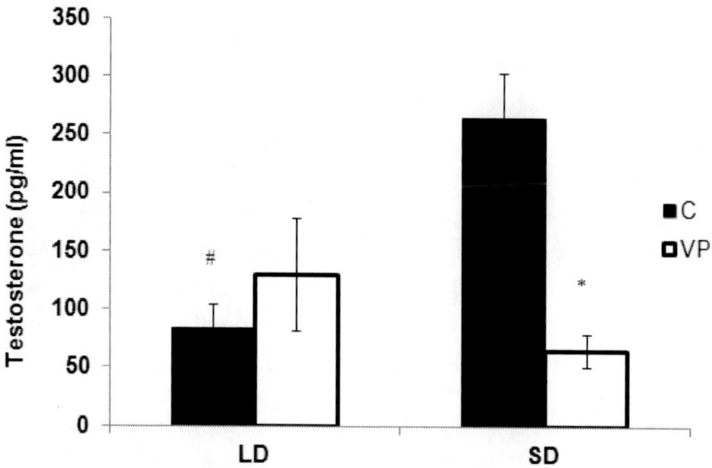

Figure 1.

In order to establish the metabolic status of the tested mice we also detected serum levels of free fatty acid (FFA) in VP treated males, compared with their control. SD-VP mice were more sensitive to VP lypolitic effect and their FFA level was increased significantly ($p<0.05$) (Table 2).

Our results show that LD-acclimated mice had significantly lower testosterone levels than SD-control mice (80 pg/ml and 250 pg/ml, respectively, $F_{1,11}=6.7$, $p<0.05$). VP treatment (VP) decreased significantly testosterone levels ($p<0.05$) in SD-acclimated mice, compared to their control group (C). (Figure 1).

A trend to increase leptin levels in SD-mice and decrease it in LD-mice was noted in response to exogenous VP treatment (VP). A correlation between gonads status and leptin plasma levels was noted. SD-VP mice showed a significant ($p<0.05$, $R^2=0.48$) positive correlation (Spearman test) between leptin serum concentration and relative testis mass (W_t) as a per cent of body weight (W_b) (Figure 2).

Modifications in aldosterone (nr3c2), and vasopressin (AVP) mRNA receptor genes expression in the gonads and in WAT as a response to VP treatment were noted. Quantification of VP receptor expression in gonads and WAT expanded our knowledge regarding the reproductive system sensitivity to VP. VP treatment (VP) decreased significantly ($p<0.05$) VP receptor genes expression (RQ: relative quantification) in testis of LD-mice, compared with control (VPc) group (Figure 3).

In SD-mice a significant ($p<0.05$) decrease in nr3c2 mRNA receptor expression (RQ: relative quantification) in testis was noted as a result of VP treatment (VP) (Figure 4).

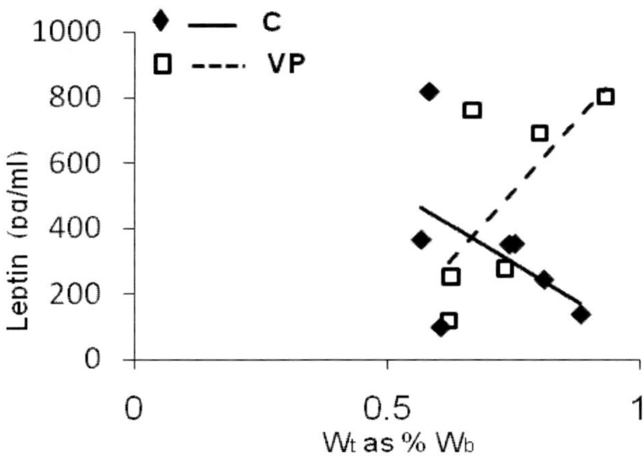

Figure 2.

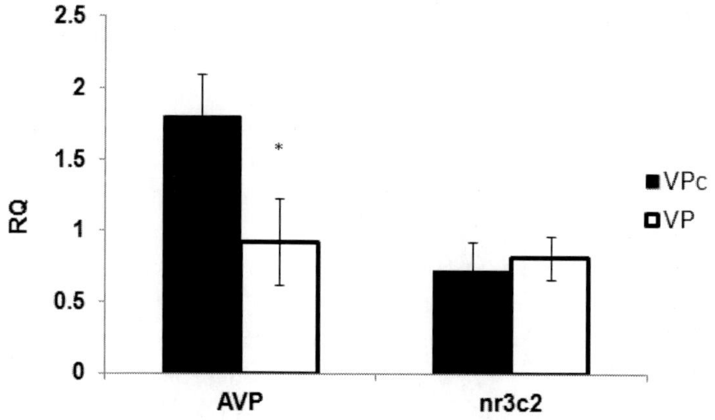

Figure 3.

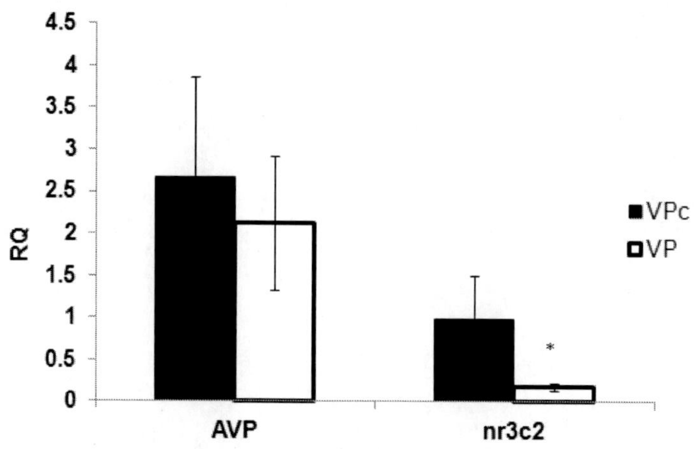

Figure 4.

A relative receptor gene expression in WAT was show a significant ($F_{1, 10}$=1.33 p<0.05) decrease in nr3c2 mRNA receptor expression (RQ: relative quantification) in SD-C–mice compared with LD-C-acclimated mice. SD-VP mice had a significant (p<0.05) increase in expression of nr3c2 mRNA receptor in WAT, compared with their control group (C-SD). Interestingly, VP treated groups had similar levels of nr3c2-receptor expression, in both SD- and LD-acclimated mice (Figure 5).

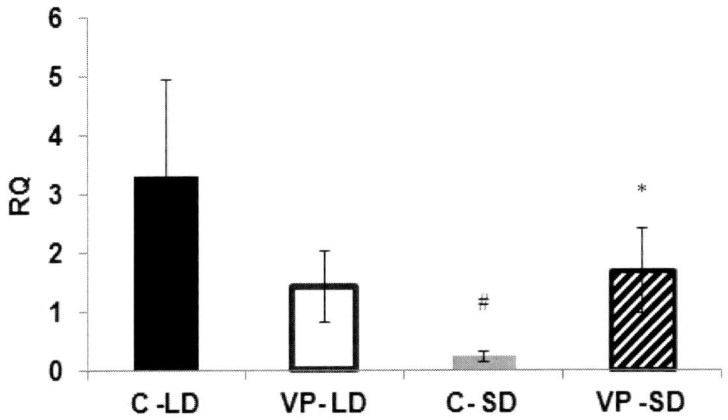

Figure 5.

DISCUSSION

The driving force in desert ecosystems is water and the intervals between episodes of water input into the ecosystem vary and in some years there may be no input at all [33]. It has been suggested that water availability can serve as a reliable cue for reproduction [46-50, 37, 38]. Water restriction was also effective in reducing reproductive activity in males of the prairie vole (*M. ochrogaster*) and in males of wild mice (*Mus musculus*) but not in the laboratory strain [48], suggesting that water availability may regulate breeding independently of photoperiod and food availability [52]. In addition to its osmoregulating function, VP affects the reproductive system [25, 30] and therefore, it was suggested as a potential candidate for transmitting the message of water shortage to the reproductive system of desert adapted rodents [37, 38, 46]. We tested the reproductive response of males from a desert adapted population of *A. cahirinus* to VP. Spermatogenesis was significantly reduced in VP-treated *A. russatus* individuals compared with their controls and compared with males from a mesic population of *A. cahirinus*, supporting this idea [39]. The results of our study show that VP treatment *per se*, caused a significant ($p<0.05$) decrease of testosterone level in SD-acclimated males, compared with their control group. The results of our study show an *in vivo* VP effect on FFA release under SD-acclimation, it caused a significant increase ($p<0.05$) in FFA release (Table 2). The suggested mechanism for such an effect was lypolisis [51].

Molecular results manifested the expression of AVP and nr3c2 mRNA receptors in testis and nr3c2 mRNA receptor in WAT, suggesting a direct effect of water on reproduction. Specific, high-affinity, low-capacity binding sites for AVP of the V1 subtype was identified in the Leydig cells of adult rat testes [53]. VP treatment resulted in a decrease of VP receptor gene expression, in LD-acclimated male testes, and a decrease in aldosterone (nr3c2) receptors gene expression in SD-acclimated males. Interestingly, nr3c2 expression levels were similar under acclimation to both photoperiods after VP treatment.

However, the existence of nr3c2 in WAT may suggest its' involvement in modulation of reproductive activity. Expression of these receptors was affected by our treatments as well as by acclimation to the different photoperiod regimes.

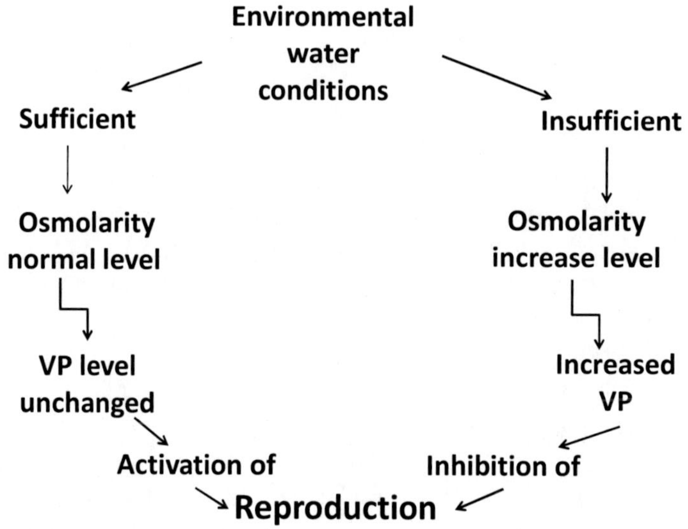

Environmental cues (availability of water) affecting reproduction in desert adapted common spiny mice *Acomys cahirinus*.

CONCLUSION

From the results of our study on reproduction and metabolism of desert-adapted males *A. cahirinus* may be concluded that more than one environmental signal is necessary for full activation of the reproductive system. As discovered in earlier studies, changes in photoperiod can be an initial signal where availability of water can serve as ultimate cues. Reproduction was affected by both, photoperiod and VP treatment.

Serum levels of testosterone were higher in SD-acclimated mice thus suggesting that mice of this population are short day breeders. However, these higher levels were significantly affected by VP while under LD-acclimation such a response was not noted. Furthermore, the testosterone response of SD-acclimated to VP treatment may indicated that if sufficient water is not available in the habitat and VP levels increase the male reproductive system may be suppressed. We observed a few significant correlations, which highlight the link between reproduction and sufficient amount of resources for maintaining metabolism.

Molecular findings supports the idea that changes in the plasma levels of VP can be picked up by testis directly or indirectly, *via* another endocrine site, such as WAT.

Our results also support the idea that different physiological systems could be integrated by a single hormonal signal. Therefore, our results support the idea of the integrated use of environmental signals for reproduction timing in desert-adapted rodent these result was also revealed on the molecular level.

REFERENCES

[1] Solomon, E., Berg, L., Martin, D. Biology, 6th edition. Brooks: Cole Publishing; 2002.

[2] Leng, G; Brown, CH; Russell, JA. Physiological pathways regulating the activity of magnocellular neurosecretory cells. *Progressive Neurobiology,* 1999, 57,625–655.

[3] Mason, W.T. (1980). Supraoptic neurones of rat hypothalamus are osmosensitive. *Nature* , 287,154–157.

[4] Bankir, L; Fernandes, S; Bardoux, P; Bouby, N; Bichet, DG. Vasopressin-V2 receptor stimulation reduces sodium excretion in healthy humans. *Journal American Society Nephrology*, 2005, 16, 1920–1928.

[5] McCormik, S.D. and Bradshow, D. (2006). Hormonal control of salt and water balance in vertebrates. *General and Comparative Endocrinology*, 147, 3-8.

[6] Bankir, L. (2001). Antidiuretic action of vasopressin: Quantitative aspects and interaction between V1a and V2 receptor-mediated effects. *Cardiovascular Research*, 51, 372-390.

[7] Birnbaumer, M. (2001). The V2 vasopressin receptor mutations and fluid homeostasis. *Cardiovascular Research*, 51, 409-415.

[8] De Kloet, E.R. (2003), Hormones, Brain and stress. *Endocrine regulations,* 37, 51-68.

[9] Hanley, MR; Benton, HP; Lightman, SL; Todd, K; Bone, EA; Fretten, P; Palmer, S; Kirk, CJ; Michell, RH. A vasopressin-like peptide in the mammalian sympathetic nervous system. *Nature,* 1984, 309, 358–261.

[10] Nussey, SS; Ang, VT; Jenkins, JS; Chowdrey, HS; Bisset, GW. Brattleboro rat adrenal contains vasopressin. *Nature,* 1984,310, 64–66.

[11] Guillon, G; Grazzini, E; Andrez, M; Breton, C; Trueba, M; Serradeil-LeGal, C; Boccara, G; Derick, S; Chouinard, L; Gallo-Payet, N. Vasopressin: a potent autocrine/paracrine regulator of mammal adrenal functions. *Endocrine Research*, 1998, 24, 703–710.

[12] Fuller, PJ; Clements, JA; Tregear, GW; Nicolaidis, I; Whitfield, PL; Funder, JW. Vasopressin-neurophysin II gene expression in the ovary: studies in Sprague-Dawley, Long-Evans and Brattleboro rats. *Journal Endocrinology,* 1985, 105, 317–321.

[13] Stones, RW; Vials, A; Milner, P; Beard, RW; Burnstock, G. Release of vasoactive agents from the isolated perfused human ovary. *Europe Journal Obstetrics Gynecology Reproductive Biology*, 1996, 67, 191–196.

[14] Kasson, BG; Meidan, R; Hsueh, AJ. Identification and characterization of arginine vasopressin-like substances in the rat testis. *Journal Biological Chemistry*, 1985, 260, 5302–5307.

[15] Fillion, C; Malassine, A; Tahri-Joutei, A; Allevard, AM; Bedin, M; Gharib, C; Hugues, JN; Pointis, G. Immunoreactive arginine vasopressin in the testis: immunocytochemical localization and testicular content in normal and experimental cryptorchid mouse. *Biological Reproduction*, 1993, 48, 786–792.

[16] Kiraly, M; Audigier, S; Tribollet, E; Barbaris, C; Dolivo, M; Dreifuss, JJ. Biochemical and electrophysiological evidence of functional vasopressin receptors in the rat superior cervical ganglion. *Proc. Natl. Acad. Sci.,* 1986, 83, 5335–5339.

[17] Grazzini, E; Lodboerer, AM; Perez-Martin, A; Joubert, D; Guillon, G. Molecular and functional characterization of V1b vasopressin receptor in rat adrenal medulla. *Endocrinology,* 1996, 137, 3906–3914.

[18] Brostrom, MA; Reilly, BA; Wilson, FJ; Brostrom, CO. Vasopressin-induced hypertrophy in H9c2 heart-derived myocytes. *Journal Biochemestry Cell Biology*, 2000, 32, 993–1006.

[19] Monstein, HJ; Truesdsson, M; Ryberg, A; Ohlsson, B. Vasopressin receptor mRNA expression in the human gastrointestinal tract. *European Surgery Research,* 2008, 40, 34–40.

[20] Gopalakrishnan, V; Triggle, CR; Sulakhe, PV; McNeill, JR. Characterization of a specific high affinity [3H] arginine 8 vasopressin-binding site on liver microsomes from different strains of rat and the role of magnesium. *Endocrinology,* 1986,118, 990–997.

[21] Schaffler, A; Binart, N; Scholmerich, J; Buchler,C. Hypothesis paper Brain talks with fat--evidence for a hypothalamic-pituitary-adipose axis? *Neuropeptides*, 2005, 39, 363-367.

[22] Austin, CR. and Short, RV. Hormonal control of reproduction. Cambridge: Cambridge University Press; 1984.

[23] Carter, CS; DeVries, AC; Getz, LL. Physiological substrates of mammalian monogamy: the prairie vole model. *Neuroscience Biobehaviour Review*, 1995, 19, 303–314.

[24] Winslow, JT; Hastings, N; Carter, CS; Harbaugh, CR; Insel, TR. A role for central vasopressin in pair bonding in monogamous prairie voles. *Nature,* 1993,365, 545–548.

[25] Wang, ZX; Liu, Y; Young, LJ; Insel, TR. Hypothalamic vasopressin gene expression increases in both males and females postpartum in a biparental rodent. *Journal Neuroendocrinology*, 2000, 12, 111 – 120.

[26] Rhodes, M.E. and Rubin, R.T. (1999). Functional sex differences ('sexual diergism') of central nervous system cholinergic systems, vasopressin, and hypothalamic–pituitary– adrenal axis activity in mammals: a selective review. *Brain Research Review*, 30,135– 52.

[27] Crofton, JT; Share, L; Brooks, DP. Pressor responsiveness to and secretion of vasopressin during the estrous cycle. *American Journal Physiology,* 1988, 255, R1041– R1048.

[28] Crofton, JT; Ratliff, DL; Brooks, DP; Share, L. The metabolic clearance rate of and pressor responses to vasopressin in male and female rats. *Endocrinology* ,1986, 118, 1777– 81.

[29] Ota, M; Crofton, JT; Liu, H; Festavan, G; Share, L. Increased plasma osmolarity stimulates peripheral and central vasopressin release in male and female rats. *American Journal Physiology*, 1994 ,267, R923–R928.

[30] Forsling, ML; Akerlund, M; Stromberg, P. Variations in plasma concentrations of vasopressin during the menstrual cycle. *Journal Endocrinology,* 1981, 89, 263– 266.

[31] Vaughan, T.A., Ryan, J.M., Czaplewski, N.J. (2000). Mammalogy. Philadelphia: Saunders College Publishing.

[32] Nelson, RJ; Dark, J; Zucker, I. Influence of photoperiod, nutrition and water availability on reproduction of male California voles (*Microtus californicus*). *Journal of reproduction and fertility*, 1983, 69, 473-477.

[33] Noy-Meir, I. (1973). Desert ecosystems: environment and producers. *Annual Review of Ecology and Systematic*, 4, 25-51.

[34] Bronson, F.H. (1989). Mammalian reproductive biology. Chicago: University of Chicago Press.

[35] Bronson, F.H. (2009). Climate change and seasonal reproduction in mammals, Philosophical transactions of the Royal Society of London. *Biological sciences, Series B*, 364 (1534), 3331-3340.

[36] Schwimmer ,H . and Haim, A.(2009). Physiological adaptations of small mammals to desert ecosystems. *Integrative Zoology* , 4, 357-366.

[37] Bukovetzky, E; Schwimmer, H; Fares, F; Haim, A. (2012a). Photoperiodicity and increasing salinity as environmental cues for reproduction in desert adapted rodents. *Hormones and Behavior*, 61, 84-90.

[38] Shanas, U. and Haim, A.(2004). Diet salinity and vasopressin as reproduction modulators in the desert-dwelling golden spiny mouse (*Acomys russatus*). *Physiology and Behavior* , 81, 645-650.

[39] Wube, T; Fares, F; Haim, A. A differential response in the reproductive system and energy balance of spiny mice *Acomys* populations to vasopressin treatment. *Comparative biochemistry and physiology*, part A, 2008, 151, 499-504.

[40] Wube, T; Haim, A; Fares, F. Effect of increased dietary salinity on the reproductive status and energy intake of xeric and mesic populations of the spiny mouse, *Acomys*, *Physiology and Behavior*, 2009, 96 , 122-127.

[41] Ahima, R.S. (2006). Metabolic actions of adipocyte hormones: focus on adiponectin. *Obesity,* 14(1), 9S–15S.

[42] Trayhurn, P. and Wood, I. S. (2004). Adipokines: inflammation and the pleiotropic role of white adipose tissue. *British Journal of Nutrition* ,92 , 347-355.

[43] Schaffler, A; Scholmerich, J; Buchler, C. The role of 'adipotropins' and the clinical importance of a potential hypothalamic-pituitary-adipose axis. Natural Clinical Practice. *Endocrinology and Metabolism* , 2006, 2, 374-383.

[44] Friedman, J.M. and Halaas, J.L. (1998). Leptin and the regulation of body weight in mammals. *Nature,* 395, 763-770.

[45] Bukovetzky, E; Fares, F; Schwimmer H; Haim ,A. Reproductive and metabolic responses of desert adapted common spiny male mice (*Acomys cahirinus*) to vasopressin treatment. *Comparative Biochemistry and Physiology*, Part A, 2012,162(4), 349-356.

[46] Bukovetzky, E; Fares, F; Haim,A. Metabolic and endocrine responses of desert-adapted Mice Reproductive System to Increased Salinity, *Journal of Life Sciences*, accepted.

[47] Nelson, R.J. (1987). Water availability affects reproduction in deer mice. *Biological Reproduction*, 37, 257–260.

[48] Nelson, R.J.(1988). Restricted water intake influences male reproduction in two strains of house mice (*Mus musculus*). *Physiological Behavior*, 43, 217– 221.

[49] Nelson, R.J.(1989). Simulated drought influences reproduction in male prairie voles. *Physiological Behavior*, 46, 849–852.

[50] Sicard, B; Fuminier, F; Maurel, D; Boissin, J. Temperature and water conditions mediate the effects of day length on the breeding cycle of a Sahelian rodent, *Arvicanthis niloticus*. *Biological Reproduction*, 1993, 49,716– 722.

[51] Vaughan, M.(1961). Effect of hormones on glucose metabolism in adipose tissue. *Journal of Biological Chemistry*, 236, 2196–2199.

[52] Nelson, RJ; Gubernick, DJ; Blom, JM. Influence of photoperiod, green food, and water availability on reproduction in male California mice (Peromyscus *californicus*). *Physiology and Behavior,* 1995, 57 (6), 1175-1180.

[53] Tahri-Joutei, A. and Pointis, G. (1989). Developmental changes in arginine vasopressin receptors and testosterone stimulation in Leydig cells. *Endocrinology,* 125, 605–611.

INDEX

A

B

C

D

E

F

G

H

I

J

K

L

M

N

O

P

Q

R

S

T

U

V

W